COMPUTERS IN THE PRACTICE OF MEDICINE VOLUME II
ISSUES IN MEDICAL COMPUTING

COMPUTERS IN THE PRACTICE OF MEDICINE VOLUME II
ISSUES IN MEDICAL COMPUTING

H. Dominic Covvey
Toronto General Hospital
Toronto, Ontario, Canada

Neil Harding McAlister
Toronto General Hospital
Toronto, Ontario, Canada

ADDISON-WESLEY PUBLISHING COMPANY

Reading, Massachusetts · Menlo Park, California
London · Amsterdam · Don Mills, Ontario · Sydney

This book is in the
Addison-Wesley Series
Computers in the Practice of Medicine

Library of Congress Cataloging in Publication Data

Covvey, H. Dominic.
    Computers in the practice of medicine.

    (Addison-Wesley series in computers in the
practice of medicine)
    Includes indexes.
    CONTENTS: vol. I. Introduction to computing con-
cepts.—vol. II. Issues in medical computing.
    1. Medicine — Data processing. I. McAlister, Neil
Harding, joint author. II. Title. III. Series.
R858.C68   001.6'4'02461   79-14099
ISBN 0-201-01251-0 (v. 1)
ISBN 0-201-01249-9 (v. 2)

ISBN 0-201-01249-9
ABCDEFGHIJ-AL-89876543210

This book is dedicated to Ken Sevcik, Derek Corneil, John Mylopoulos, Ron Baecker, and all our other friends in Computer Science at the University of Toronto.

Preface

Health professionals are becoming increasingly aware of the importance of computers in their work, and they are often acutely aware that their training has done little to prepare them to approach the rapidly expanding field of medical computing in a knowledgeable way.

The books in this series attempt to provide the health-care worker with some of this missing information. These books are written for physicians, hospital administrators, nurses, laboratory technologists, medical students, and others whose main interest is in the health-care field. Their goal is to give such readers sufficient knowledge to make them comfortable with computer systems, current computer technology, and some of the more important issues in medical computing. The reader who masters this material should be able both to listen intelligently and to talk sensibly about the computer. These books might best be viewed not as "cookbook" approaches to medical computing but as "working papers" that outline the basics, review the state of the art, identify typical problem areas, and offer practical suggestions for coping with these problems.

The first volume in this series, *Computers in the Practice of Medicine, Vol. I—Introduction to Computing Concepts,* described computing machinery and elementary concepts of software to a computer-naive health-care professional.

However, an understanding of the "nuts and bolts" of computer technology, although an essential prerequisite for anyone involved in medical computing, is far from sufficient background. Equally important is an appreciation of several major issues affecting the practice of medical computing.

This, the second volume in the Addison-Wesley series on medical computing, discusses these important issues, so vital to the success of any medical-computing venture. The first chapter provides a brief overview of the problems. The second chapter attempts to convince the reader that due consideration of these issues is a necessity. Subsequently, the topics of software engineering, human engineering, privacy and security, cost analysis, functional specifications and contracts, system development, management, and the education of both medical-computing specialists and consumers of their services are considered in detail.

Chapter 12 integrates all of these issues in a practical discussion of how all of them together will need to be considered as part of a funding application. Anyone who has submitted grant applications for funding for a medical-computing project is aware that financial support is not automatically forthcoming. These days, such requests for funding are usually sent to experts for review, and the panel of referees increasingly includes specialists in medical computing. Scientists who seek other people's money in support of their medical-computing schemes will have to *convince* reviewers of the feasability of their proposals. Therefore, in this chapter we review each of the issues that has been discussed in previous chapters in the context of a formal grant application, written with an eye to quality, reviewability, and therefore fundability.

The final chapter examines current trends in hardware and software technology and indulges in some speculation about where medical computing is going in the future.

This particular book is aimed not just at health-care professionals but also at computer scientists who are working in a medical context. Most computer science education is slanted toward the needs of the business community: Only a few institutions of higher learning provide formal courses on medical informatics. Thus many computer scientists who have to work as medical-computing experts are left without specific training for the unique constraints and problems of the medical environment. We sincerely hope that the observations in this book may be of help to such readers.

ACKNOWLEDGMENTS

We would again like to express our gratitude to all of the people who have directly or indirectly contributed to this work.

Professor George Torrance of the School of Business, McMaster University, co-authored Chapter 6 with us, and we appreciate his help. Thanks also go to our research assistant, Ms. Maeve ("the Slaeve") O'Beirne, and to Ms. Debbie Schreiber, who continues to astonish us by typing completed manuscript pages as fast as we can produce them.

Again, we are most grateful to Dr. E. Douglas Wigle for his continuing support of this project. Of course, we have benefited from the professional skills and personal support of our editors, Mr. Bill Gruener and Ms. Mary Clare McEwing, and from many other people at Addison-Wesley. And finally, special thanks go to our families.

It should go without saying that all the people who have helped us in this effort are exempt from blame for any errors or omissions in it.

Toronto   N. H. M.
February 1980   H. D. C.

Contents

III

WHY ARE THERE ISSUES?

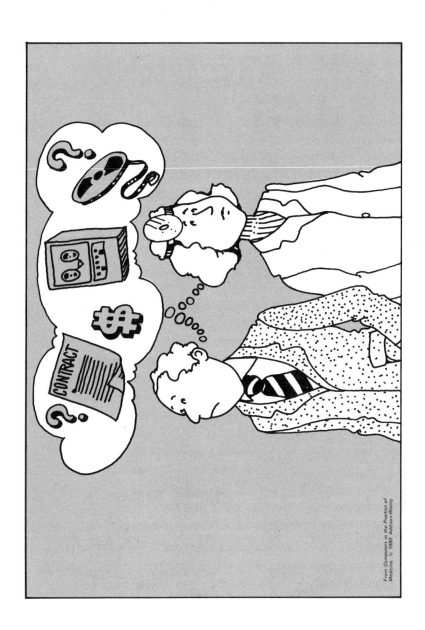

1

Overview: What are the Issues?

The Shepherd To His Love

Come live with me and be my love,
And we will all the pleasures prove
That hills and valleys, dale and field,
And all the craggy mountains yield.

There will we sit upon the rocks
And see the shepherds feed their flocks,
By shallow rivers, to whose falls
Melodious birds sing madrigals.

There will I make thee beds of roses
And a thousand fragrant posies,
A cap of flowers, and a kirtle
Embroidered all with leaves of myrtle.

A gown made of the finest wool,
Which from our pretty lambs we pull,
Fair lined slippers for the cold,
With buckles of the purest gold.

Thy silver dishes for thy meat
As precious as the gods do eat
Shall on an ivory table be
Prepared each day for thee and me.

The shepherd swains shall dance and sing
For they delight each May-morning:
If these delights thy mind may move,
Then live with me and be my love.

                              Christopher Marlowe

The Nymph's Reply

If all the world were fair and young,
And truth in every shepherd's tongue,
These pretty pleasures might me move
To live with thee, and be thy love.

But Time drives flocks from field to fold,
When rivers rage and rocks grow cold;
And Philomel becometh dumb;
The rest complain of cares to come.

The flowers do fade, and wanton fields
To wayward Winter reckoning yields:
A honey tongue, a heart of gall,
Is fancy's spring, but sorrow's fall.

Thy gowns, thy shoes, thy beds of roses,
Thy cap, thy kirtle, and thy posies,
Soon break, soon wither, —soon forgotten,
In folly ripe, in reason rotten.

But could youth last, and love still breed,
Had joys no date, nor age no need,
Then these delights my mind might move
To live with thee and be thy love.

Sir Walter Raleigh

The seductive call of automation sounds sweet to the ears of
the medical community and of hospital administrators. Until
recently, health professionals have been used to the "silver dishes"
and "ivory tables" afforded by unrestricted budgets, and they have
acquired a taste for expensive technology. It is now virtually
taken for granted that clinical judgment alone will be insufficient to
establish a diagnosis or to determine appropriate treatment for most
patients. Given a marketplace full of people who already believe in
progress through technology, it is not surprising that entrepreneurs
with financial interest in the dissemination of computers should be
eager to woo health-care workers with sweet refrains about the

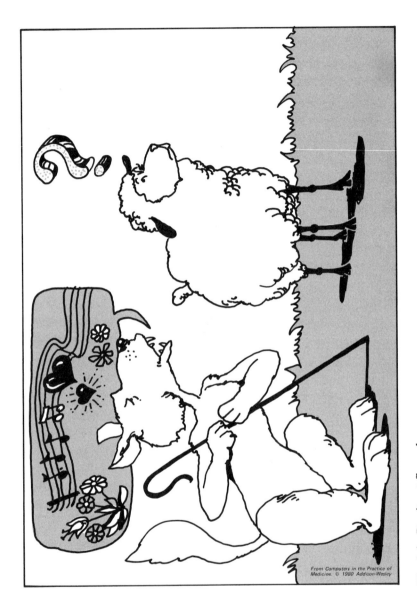

Fig. 1.1. Don't get fleeced
Be wary of uncritical acceptance of other people's claims about computers!

pleasures of automation — the ultimate in technological progress (Fig. 1.1).

Even as the nymph takes a skeptical view of the rosy picture painted by her shepherd swain, so should we be wary of uncritical acceptance of other people's claims about computers, for many an automation scheme has proved to be "in folly ripe, in reason rotten."

Healthy skepticism does not imply a negative, cynical attitude. It does imply, however, a serious effort on the part of all nymphs to evaluate the honeyed claims of shepherds with computers to sell.

Fortunately, there are several distinct issues in medical computing that can be addressed separately and that can give structure to the evaluation. Each of these issues will be considered in depth in subsequent chapters. For now, though, let's get a brief overview.

FUNDING MEDICAL COMPUTING

There is a very practical reason why anyone who becomes involved in medical computing should be interested in all of these issues: Sooner or later they will have to convince some funding agency to give them money to support their plans.

Many granting agencies have been "stung" by ill-conceived medical-computing projects that they have supported. Now that they have learned their lessons the hard way, they are less likely to open the purse strings for poorly justified medical-computing schemes. Increasingly, applications for funds for medical computing are sent to medical-computing specialists for review. These reviewers will be totally unimpressed by grandiose claims of what might be achieved with the mere input of money. What they want to see is that the sponsors of such research have duly considered the practical, problematic issues at stake in their proposed projects, and that they have developed strategies for anticipating such problems or for coping with them if they occur.

As you read the following chapters, bear in mind that these important issues should be dealt with in your next funding application for a medical-computing project. There is nothing theoretical or "philosophical" about this: Those who ignore the issues will soon be financially left out in the cold, their ignorance bared for the world — or, at least, for the reviewers — to see.

TECHNICAL ISSUES

Software Engineering

One of the most vexing issues in medical computing is perhaps one of the least obvious, that of software engineering. To the uninitiated, it is not self-evident that there are many ways of "skinning a cat" in computer programming. Furthermore, some ways are significantly better than others.

Programs that are written in a "quick and dirty" fashion, that are written in low-level languages, or that are undocumented may leave an inscrutable legacy to future generations of programmers who may be called on to change them.

And change is often required — not only because the first shot at a program often misses the mark, but also because errors in programming may become apparent only after weeks, months, or occasionally years of routine use of a program. Only the naive assume that a computer program works perfectly. It is not possible to *prove* the correctness of most programs. The best that can usually be done is to test them thoroughly, and there are formal techniques for doing this. However, many programs are pushed into active service without adequate testing. Latent "bugs" may lie dormant in segments of seldom-executed code, only to emerge much later.

Most users of a computer system may not be experts in software engineering, but they should be aware of its importance in order to appreciate the necessity of acquiring competent help before buying or writing programs. Programs must be selected or written as carefully as hardware is chosen, and they should be examined not simply on the basis of what they do but on how they do it. Chapter 3 introduces the basics about the "how."

Human Engineering

The commitment to automation often implies a substantial restructuring of an organization. Businesspeople often work with computers at arm's length, through an intermediary. In medicine, however, physicians, nurses, and other health-care personnel work directly with the computer in a "hands-on" situation. They are therefore intimately interested in how the machine works for them. Complex, obscure, or unnecessarily difficult-to-use computer systems can be a genuine hardship to the medical-computer user. Human engineering, the art of making systems easier to use, is therefore an essential ingredient in the development of any medical-computing scheme.

In any working environment, medicine included, those who have wished to introduce new procedures, new forms, or new data collection methods have always been aware that they are, in essence, disrupting the way in which their colleagues conduct their business. Computers represent a somewhat more grand and sweeping means of disrupting current practice. However, they bring another danger with them: They may make future change quantitatively and qualitatively more difficult.

Human engineering and the impact of computers on the human clinical environment will be examined in Chapter 4.

Privacy and Security

A great deal has been written about the privacy and security of computer records, probably because it is an area about which it is easy to say something — although seldom something significant. There is an aura of white knights in shining armor around those who preach that personal data must be protected from unauthorized, prying eyes. However, having paid lavish lip service to this "motherhood-and-apple-pie issue," one is faced with a much more difficult task in trying to *do* something about it. The average medical-computer installation is woefully lacking in even elementary physical security precautions against vandalism and fire. Thus we compartmentalize our "concern" into things we believe in and publicly crow about, and things we are willing to spend money on in order to achieve a useful result.

Without a doubt, the advent of automation threatens health care with several new and substantial privacy and security problems. The relative ease with which computer-stored information can be organized and retrieved makes it much less difficult to find things that were once scattered diffusely in many paper medical records. Without actually stealing anything tangible, an unauthorized party can sometimes invade a computer system over the telephone and make an illegal copy of the desired data. The ability to transmit data between systems poses an even more ominous problem: It is now possible to collate data from two or more separate databases in order to piece together information that would not be available from any one separate data source. Finally, the extreme miniaturization of stored records realized through automated data-recording methods makes the physical theft of computer-based information potentially much more damaging than the theft of paper charts in the past. A crook who steals one magnetic tape might get the equivalent of several dump trucks full of paper charts!

Despite the new threats to privacy and security that medical automation may pose, the issue did not originate with the advent of automation. Privacy and security of data have always been important in medicine. The computer, then, focuses our attention on some old problems and increases the urgency of solving them. We can no longer be comfortable in sweeping this issue under the rug!

We will address this issue in Chapter 5.

Economics

Because money for medical care is becoming less freely available, we are being faced with the necessity of considering the cost-justification of innovations. Everybody knows that computers are expensive. However, few have cared to examine in detail how much money they have spent on computers and how much money they save (if any) by using them. Terms such as "cost-benefit" are flung about in the absence of formal cost-benefit analysis. Expressions like "cost-effectiveness" are used in flagrant defiance of the fact that medicine still cannot agree on precise definitions of clinical "effectiveness" unless there is something as dramatic as mortality statistics involved.

An understanding of cost-justification analysis should be an integral part of the mental set of any health-care worker who is contemplating the use of a computer system. We will provide an introduction to this important area in Chapter 6.

Functional Specifications and Contracts

These are both economic and legal issues. Too many computers are purchased or leased for medical purposes in the complete absence of written agreements of any kind. Very few medical-computing systems are acquired on the basis of an enforceable contract guaranteeing their performance relative to some specification. In many cases, hidden costs and extras will add considerably to an original imprecise quotation. In the worst cases, hardware and software simply fail to perform as a vendor promised they would or as a user thought they would. The difference in the "understanding" of what a system is supposed to do as viewed by the user and by the supplier can be as great as the difference between night and day in the absence of written functional specifications to which both have agreed and in the absence of the contract that formalizes the agreement.

Such an important issue can no longer be ignored by health-care professionals who work within constrained budgets that cannot cover the cost of spectacular failure. We detail the considerations in a functional specification in Chapter 7.

MANAGEMENT ISSUES
Managing System Development

Successful applications don't just happen: They are made. When outside system developers are employed to aid in a medical-computing project, the users or their advocates are well advised to have some idea of the nature of the development process. In the case of in-house system development, effective management of the development process is an essential ingredient if an application is to be completed successfully, on time, and within planned budgetary constraints. There is a great deal more involved in project management than merely hiring a programmer and hoping for the best! Precisely what is involved will be considered in Chapter 8.

Organizing for Automation

Chapter 9 addresses the sometimes thorny problems associated with the institutional management of medical-computing endeavors. The radically different requirements of hospital business computing for administrative purposes, and medical-research computing in support of individual research projects, make separation of responsibilities essential to successful computer implementation in either field.

The overlapping concerns of the medical community and hospital administration in the area of computer services to patients make some effective and clearly understood management approach mandatory for institutional peace.

The means by which the end users of medical-computing facilities can promote and defend their own interests are also given consideration in this chapter.

EDUCATIONAL ISSUES

Training Medical-Computing Specialists

It takes a special kind of individual to take effective responsibility for a medical-computing project. The sort of person required has the ability to bridge a wide gap between computer science and health care. Many medical-computing projects have foundered precisely because their proponents were unable to find anyone to bridge this gap adequately.

Increasingly, the health care community is acknowledging the role of data processing in its affairs, and therefore there is a growing demand for medical-computing specialists. A few institutions of higher learning are beginning to respond to this perceived need, and in Chapter 10 we will look carefully at the ways in which this educational need might be met.

Conspicuous Computing: Consumer Education

Not only medical-computing specialists but also the consumers of medical computing need to be educated. It is no accident that we often feel differently about computer technology than we do about any other kind of technology that is used in medicine. What is it about computers that makes them different?

To a large extent, computers have been *oversold* both by commercial interests and by some user advocates as a general solution to all problems. There are not too many informed consumers left who believe that a computer can be put to work on their behalf by merely addressing it "O Mighty Computer!" However, there are many — too many — health-care workers who believe that it is possible to program a computer to do almost any crazy thing they can imagine. A great deal of the blame for this unreasonable level of expectation must fall squarely on the shoulders of the computer industry itself. The advertisements for medical-computer systems for every area from radiology departments to the physician's office are long on promises and pretty pictures, but short on performance specifics.

The principle at work here is what we call "conspicuous computing" [1] — an irrational lust for the aura of sophistication and progress that a person, department, or institution can acquire by becoming "computerized." The techniques of consumer motivation — that is, creating artificial needs that were not previously felt — have been just as effective in selling medical-computing products as they have been in selling automobiles. We will examine this phenomenon in some detail in Chapter 11.

QUO VADIS?
The Future of Medical Computing

Each of the issues that must be examined in an evaluation of the impact of computers on the medical environment has a "prehistory" extending well back into the precomputer era. If we remember this fact, we will be less likely to be cowed by what is only another way of doing many of the things that we have been doing for years without computer assistance. Indeed, a noted computer scientist and philosopher, Joseph Weizenbaum, has pointed out that computers are *conservative* influences as often as they are harbingers of change. [2] Could it be, for instance, that in medicine, computers have come along just in time to save our hopelessly large and inefficient medical record departments, when in fact the whole system should have been rethought and redone?

On the other hand, there is a better-than-even chance that computers will continue to provide an ever-increasing variety of valuable services to medical care — services that could not be rendered in any other way. It seems likely, for example, that profound advances in medically related artificial intelligence techniques may soon be upon us, with subsequent breakthroughs in computer-assisted diagnosis and treatment planning. In the more distant future, it may be possible that the Bionic Man and the Bionic Woman of science-fiction fame may approach reality. Who knows?

In the final chapter, therefore, we indulge in some crystal ball gazing in an effort to see where all of this intense effort in medical computing will take us within our lifetimes.

WHO CARES?

Why are all these issues important to the average user? It is very tempting to pass off discussion of these problems as mere philosophy in a headlong rush to "get on with the job" and produce — if not the perfect computer system — at least a real computer system. Such an attitude, although understandable, is dangerous. Many a *real* medical-computing system has ended in a *real* fiasco. Everyone who works in medical computing is aware of at least as many failures as successes. Naturally, the successes find their way into print. Even many of the failures are the subjects of technical papers that carefully hide the extent of the failure, while proudly describing the scope of the limited "success" that was achieved, thus making a virtue out of a frustrating necessity. The health-care worker who is contemplating his or her first brush with automation may thereby receive a misleading impression about the usefulness of computers and the ease with which they can be employed.

Nothing could be more deceiving. Computers are still difficult to use, and they can be tamed only by skilled professionals. Mere technical know-how is not enough to ensure success. Knowledge of the issues involved in medical computing is essential to achieving worthwhile results.

Why?

If computers could write their own programs, then software engineering would not be an issue. If all health-care workers found computer systems easy to use and helpful to their normal way of doing business, then human engineering would be unimportant. If we could trust everyone to respect the privacy of sensitive, personal medical data and if computers were invulnerable to fire and other natural catastrophes, then perhaps there would be no security issue. If computers were inexpensive, then the study of economic issues would be superfluous. If no one had ever lost his shirt to an unscrupulous computer vendor or if no one had ever bought the wrong computer through simple ignorance, then functional specifications and contracts would be a waste of time. If computers could set their own priorities, fund themselves, and keep all of their users happy without human intervention, then management issues would not exist. If the work force were full of medical-computing specialists and if advertising were not both insidious and effective, then the education of medical-computing specialists and of consumers would not trouble us.

But — lack-a-day! — all the world is not fair and young, nor is truth in every shepherd's tongue. Therefore, those who dismiss the issues involved in medical computing as mere philosophy do so at their own risk.

But don't simply take our word for it: The importance of proceeding with an eye to the issues is perhaps best illustrated by the sad tale of a specific case in which many of them were ignored. Because you are unlikely to read about a medical-computing failure anywhere else, one of these authors would like to share with you a tale of woe about one of his medical-computing projects that never really got off the ground. If after reading the next chapter you still maintain that the issues outlined here are for philosophers, then good luck to you! However, on with the story —

NOTES

1. N. H. McAlister and H. D. Covvey, Conspicuous computing: or, if there are users there must be pushers. *Can. Med. Assoc. J.* 116:183, 1977.

2. J. Weizenbaum, *Computer Power and Human Reason.* San Francisco: W. H. Freeman, 1976.

2

A Tale of Woe

Wherein we Defcribe the Lugubriouf Hiftorie of a Failure in Medical Computing

Once upon a time in a big hospital there was a strong mandate to create an information system for psychiatric in-patients and out-patients. It was recognized that this was an ambitious project, so it was decided that it would focus first on the support of psychiatric research on an in-patient population.

It took a full year to develop a formal proposal. It was then found that Psychiatry could not get any funds to support its brain-child. Research funding agencies called it service. The hospital budget committee called it research. Falling between two stools and failing to secure a funding commitment is the "tragic flaw" in our dramatic plot. At the time, the closely affiliated Department of Psychology's Psychophysiology Laboratory wanted to establish a computer facility for signal processing to support its own physiology research. Unlike the psychiatric database proposal, Psychophysiology managed to find some money to fund its computer system. It was therefore decided to pool the computing interests (unrelated as they were) of the Psychophysiology Lab and the Department of Psychiatry. The psychiatric database was going to get its start on the back of the psychophysiology computing system.

Although Psychophysiology had enough money for a small real-time computing system to support its experiments (a PDP-11/40 with a 2.5 Mb cartridge disk drive, and analog-to-digital hardware costing $40,000), the cost of the database-system hardware (including one disk drive of at least 50 Mb, tape drives, and communications equipment) and of the software needed to support a psychiatric database was unfortunately in the neighborhood of $100,000 to $150,000. Still at least $60,000 to $90,000 shy of the database system, Psychiatry went looking for other users who might contribute to developing a computer system that would serve information storage and retrieval functions.

Cardiology (well . . . the heart and the mind are supposed to go together!) was also looking for a computer to perform ECG analysis. They were persuaded to invest in a combined computer facility with Psychophysiology, and Cardiology therefore donated an additional $50,000 to the computer facility, some of which was used to buy a second cartridge disk — only another 2.5 Mb.

At this point, a computer system that had originally been conceived as a psychiatric database facility was now firmly dedicated to two real-time signal analysis applications — psychophysiology experiments and ECG analysis. The entire purpose of the computing system — and consequently its very design — had drastically changed from the original proposal for the psychiatric information system to a signal processing facility. Ninety thousand dollars had already been spent in total, but it had been spent on a real-time computing system. Vital hardware and software components for the *database* system were still lacking. This would have been an excellent point for the psychiatric database proponents to throw in the towel, but . . . (back to the ranch!)

There was still neither enough mass storage nor software to support the psychiatric database management system, so the facility went looking for more money. It was not difficult to find more users, but it was difficult to find *paying* users. An additional $17,000 was obtained from a research grant (this money was absorbed in simply making the system able to handle multiple users); $15,000 was contributed by the Psychology Department (which wanted to use the computer for scoring and interpreting psychological tests); and $10,000 was added to the pot (mostly for another 2.5 Mb disk) by an outside agency that wanted to use the computer system to store data on psychiatric out-patients. (At last there was a file storage and retrieval system for psychiatric patients — even though it was small enough for a 2.5 Mb disk!)

At this point, $126,000 had been spent on computer hardware and software. However, much of this money had been spent to develop a real-time computing system, not a database system. A lot of money was still needed to turn the computing system into a full-scale database facility!

At least $30,000 was needed for a reasonable-capacity disk drive of 50 Mb or more, and two of them would have been better. Further price tags included at least $10,000 more for a tape drive and another $10,000 for appropriate database management software. But there never was any money to buy these things. Thus, on top of the $126,000 already paid out, between $50,000 and $80,000 was *still* needed. Remember, a basic database system would have cost only $100,000–$150,000 in the first place.

At least it was easy to fund the diligent programming staff: Their salaries were available, unlike funds for capital equipment. The programmers could do something about the lack of software, so they labored away to create at least some database software and other programs, some of which were already commercially available, but for which funds did not exist. They were "reinventing the wheel" because the computer facility could not afford to buy existing commercial software. To add to their woes (and this is a frequent "story within a story" in this area), the programmers were faced with a complete revision of the computer's operating system and of the programming language by the company that had originally supplied it. The revised operating system and FORTRAN were very different from the originals, and they had drastic effects on existing applications software, most of which had to be rewritten.

To make matters worse still, the facility had no money for ordinary operating costs. In desperation, the facility turned to the hospital administration, which agreed to pay for half of an annual hardware maintenance contract *if employee health records were kept on the "psychiatry" computer.* This ploy was the administrative camel's nose in the psychiatric computing tent — an omen of worse things to come.

And so it went. Among other interests, Surgery wanted to climb aboard the computing bandwagon with an arrangement to keep some surgical records on the system in exchange for a small amount of funding. At this late date, some sense prevailed and Surgery was turned down. However, the Pulmonary Function Lab was brought in on the action, and pulmonary function test reporting was implemented quite successfully.

But the bastard system, conceived in an unholy union of drastically conflicting interests, failed to serve most of its users particularly well. As a psychiatric database facility it was unsuccessful because there never had been any money directed specifically to that purpose. To be sure, $126,000 had been found, but it had been found for other computing purposes. The computing facility lacked enough continuing financial backing to meet even ordinary maintenance costs.

Hospital administration moved in for the kill. It cut the salaries of the computing staff, and ultimately took over 100-percent control of the computer system because it felt that it could make use of the facility — yes indeed, that is what they thought . . .

The punchline is — you guessed it — that administration is now caught in the web, and they are beginning to realize that signal processing and accounts receivable have a "few" differences. At last report they were renting the facility to a research group. The house that Jack built has many doors: Unfortunately, most of them lead *out* — something that each user appears to learn after paying the entrance fee. Have you ever heard the old joke about the traveling salesman?

Sic transit gloria computoris!

There, in a simplified nutshell, is the sad tale of one unsuccessful medical-computing installation. It generated a few papers and even a few partially satisfied customers. But it was still a failure.

What can be learned from this fiasco, four years in the making?

The most obvious lesson is that no matter how hard you ignore the economic issues, they catch up with you anyway. Because of hopeless financial constraints, this project, like many other medical-computing endeavors that fall miserably short of original goals, was doomed in an impossible fight for survival.

Although this project was strapped by economics, it was not a cheap fiasco. In addition to the $126,000 spent on hardware and software, $200,000 was spent on salaries over a four-year period, $52,000 on maintenance of hardware and software, and $20,000 on paper forms and other expendables. In round figures, this mess cost about $400,000, and that was nowhere near enough to guarantee an effective return for the large investment.

Put simply, there is often no money to support the best intentions of those who want to become involved in medical computing. They are therefore compelled to seek the support of outside interests in order to generate a "critical mass" so that hardware, software, and support personnel can be afforded. But the wider a computer installation casts its nets to serve more and more users with unrelated interests, the more inexorably hardware, software, and human capacity fall behind increasing demands. The more you try to do, the bigger the system required to do it. When it is impossible to afford a small system to do one job, it will almost surely be impossible to afford a more expensive system to do several jobs!

In the blinding light of the retrospectoscope, not only economic issues but management issues were ignored in this facility. The original purpose and the original proposal for a computer system was to establish a psychiatric database system. There should have been a firm stand on this specification. As soon as Psychophysiology came along with its own funding, Psychophysiology should have been encouraged to establish its own specification and to seek to develop its own separate resources — not as a means of supporting the database project, but as a legitimate end in itself. From the database point of view, this experience simply proved the truism that you cannot get more than you are willing to pay for. The moment one starts prostituting one's computing goals for the sake of money, the battle is already lost. To attempt to establish a database management system with no money is ludicrous. (See Fig. 2.1.)

Several more positive lessons were learned. It was found that a pulmonary function report generator can be developed cheaply. It was learned that a minicomputer has incredible capacity and that even a diversity of mismatched applications such as the ones outlined here could not saturate it. Another way of looking at this would be to say that the facility made the same mistakes with $100,000 worth of hardware that some people have made with $1,000,000 systems.

Some interesting points about software engineering and about the people who write programs were also learned the hard way. One cannot mix database and real-time environments because most programmers are not good at both kinds of applications. Furthermore, software packages developed by other amateur users are best avoided. One particular communications software package was purchased from another university: It was undocumented and unsupported. Three months of programming effort were wasted in attempting to make it work. Eventually, the equivalent commercial communications package was bought from an established company, and it worked the first day. Penny wisdom is often pound foolishness.

This project demonstrated painfully why medical bosses enjoy low esteem among many computer scientists. Too often one forgets

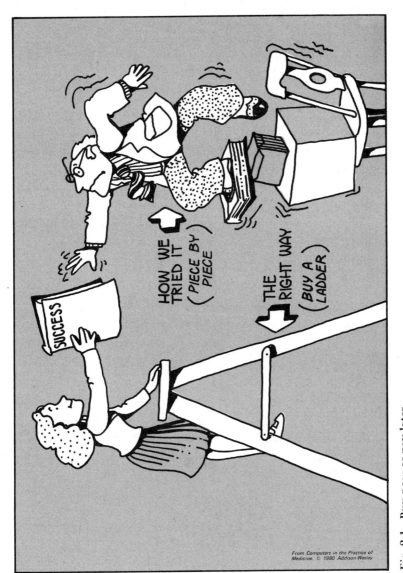

Fig. 2.1. Buy now or pay later
To reach success, you need a sensible plan. The plan may cost of lot of money, but —
Proceeding haphazardly "on the cheap" usually ends in a disaster, sometimes more expensive than
doing it the right way in the first place would have been.

that programmers are people with feelings. Writing a computer program is a creative act. If one requires a programmer to spend many months in developing a functioning program and then pulls out of a project and never implements that program, the person who created it is going to be offended. For such a reason, one of the programmers in this project resigned even before funding for his position was cut off, vowing never to work in the medical environment again. (He's now in industry.) If medicine makes a habit of throwing away experienced data processing personnel, not much progress in medical computing can be expected.

In summary, then, this tale of woe demonstrates how disregard of the important issues in medical computing can prevent the success of a project. It is therefore evident that those who dismiss these problem areas as mere philosophy do so at their own peril!

Requiescat in pace.

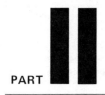

PART **II**

TECHNICAL ISSUES

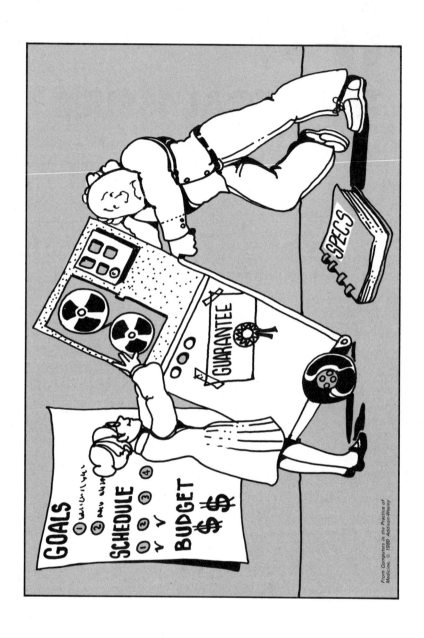

3

Software Engineering

One of the most critical issues that affects the users of computer systems is one that users are least likely to understand — software engineering. "Software engineering" refers to the use of formal methodologies for designing, writing, and testing computer programs (software). Users of a medical-computing system might wonder why such techniques should concern them. In an atmosphere in which users think of computers as mysterious "black boxes" that automatically accept input and correctly produce the required output, concern over software engineering might well appear to be superfluous. Such an atmosphere, however, is dangerous and totally unrealistic, since the issue of software engineering has an overwhelming impact on the schedule, budget, and even the success and long-term survivability of a medical-computing endeavor.

A computer program that is flung together with primary regard to expediency, with little concern for sound design and less for producing a testable product, bears a relationship to proper software that is roughly analogous to the relationship between chicken coops and houses. Both chicken coops and houses fall under the generic term "buildings," but the latter can be a home fit for a king, while the former may barely keep the rain off the chickens! "Chicken house programming," like "chicken house carpentry," results in a low-quality product that is not fit for the consumer.

Unfortunately for many naive users, the weaknesses of inferior programming may not be immediately recognizable to the untrained eye, and the results of sloppy work may not manifest themselves until long after the unscrupulous builder has absconded with the user's money or the unskillful worker has departed. The principle of *caveat emptor* applies here, and buyers are well advised to inform themselves of the features that distinguish programming expertise from slipshod approaches that may, in the long run, be more expensive, if not fatal to their applications.

WHY ENGINEER SOFTWARE?

The bottom line of software development is economics. As we stressed in the first volume in this series, software development is the most expensive component of a computer system, often exceeding hardware costs by a factor of two or more. [1]

Software development is expensive because it takes so long to produce finished programs that work according to specifications. There are four separate phases in creating useful software: design, coding, testing, and maintenance. These four phases, and estimates of the amount of time that is commonly devoted to each, are outlined in an excellent paper by Zelkowitz. [2]

In the *design* phase, someone must identify the problem that needs to be solved by automation and then develop an appropriate programming strategy for solving that problem. Zelkowitz estimates that in larger applications, this phase may account for about 11 percent of the entire software development effort.

The second phase of the process — *coding* — is that activity that people commonly think of as "programming": the actual writing of statements in some programming language. But to view coding as the main effort of "programming" is quite misleading, since this activity may account for as little as seven percent of total software development effort in a large application.

Once code has been written, *testing* it may account for another 15 percent of the time spent in creating software.

According to Zelkowitz, a whopping 67 percent of the time and money expended on creating a large software system is accounted for by the fourth and final phase of the process — *software maintenance.* The unhappy fact remains that it is impossible to detect all or even most errors in a program that *appears* to be functioning properly. Many errors will become apparent only after a program has been in use for weeks, months, or occasionally even years. As each of these errors announces itself, it must be corrected; thus program modifications become necessary. Additionally, user requirements in a given application change constantly, and users' changing needs will necessitate periodic software modifications.

Not only is software development expensive, but also, unfortunately, there is no assurance of its ultimate success. The large investment, both of time and of money, in hardware acquisition and software development does not pay off in terms of useful results until software is designed, written, tested, debugged, and found to be working correctly. If for any reason the programming process halts short of the intended software product, the entire investment is a loss. When problems are encountered in software development, deadlines are missed, budgets are exceeded, priorities change, and the results may be a large commitment for very little practical return. In such circumstances, it has not been uncommon to see desperate sponsors "throwing good money after bad" in order to salvage something worthwhile out of a programming fiasco.

Anything that could reduce the risk in software development and that could help to assure the favorable outcome of the process would be desirable. However, the inherent limitations of the programming process severely restrict the potential for instituting any such procedures.

An interesting constant in software development has been discovered: When all four phases of the development process are considered, it would appear that a programmer working alone produces, on the average, fewer than twenty lines of tested, working code per day. [3] This low figure reflects the enormous proportion of the programmer's time that must be spent in testing and in software maintenance. Since many programs routinely run into hundreds, or even a couple of thousand of lines of code, the total output of user-ready software that one programmer can produce in a year is not large.

Often in a medical environment, time is an important consideration in software develoment. Once a need has been perceived, a medical-research goal, a patient-care priority, or an administrative plan may demand rapid implementation. For instance, a two-year development period could render needs obsolete before they had ever been met. The necessity to conduct several projects simultaneously or a very large project within a reasonable amount of time, will demand the addition of extra programming staff in a medical-computing laboratory.

Unfortunately, when two or more programmers work on the same project, the time-saving realized is not directly proportional to the number of programmers. In fact, (as has been pointed out by Brooks and Zelkowitz), adding more programmers to a team also introduces more problems of communication among the programmers as they attempt to coordinate their efforts, and this necessary communication occupies an increasingly large segment of each programmer's time. [4] Zelkowitz estimates that if one programmer is capable of writing a 5000-line program in a year, five programmers working in a team could produce only 20,000 lines of code per year — and not 25,000 lines, as we might have expected. The bigger the team, the less efficient it is. This fact is a limitation that bedevils larger programming projects.

Since a programmer's productivity in lines of code is about the same no matter what programming language is used, it makes sense to employ high-level programming languages with powerful statements, rather than low-level assembler-type languages. [5]

However, no matter what language is used, the cost per statement is very high. It makes sense to do everything possible to obtain the highest quality software in return for this big investment. In an effort to minimize errors, maximize program efficiency, and reduce testing and software maintenance time to a minimum, the discipline of software engineering has developed. This discipline is predicated on the observation that a formally *designed* piece of software is more likely to approach perfection more quickly than an equivalent program that has been thrown together by old-fashioned ad hoc methods.

To most health-care workers, even the elementary concepts of computers and computer programming may be mysterious. To such readers we recommend the first volume in this series, which deals with these general, introductory concepts in a simple way. Once the basics have been grasped, the computer system user is in a position to look more closely at the four phases of software development, to which we now turn.

THE DESIGN PHASE

Details of the various techniques that have been developed for software design are beyond the scope of this book. Here we will enumerate a few of the more common methods only briefly: Interested readers can find greater depth in the references listed at the end of the chapter. They should realize, of course, that entire university courses are devoted to this subject.

One of the better-known techniques is variously called *top down development,* or simply *structured programming.* Basically, this technique is a method of structuring and analyzing a problem in a progressively refined manner, from the highest or most abstract level down to the lowest or most detailed level, progressively adding more and more detail to the subsystems, the structures, or the modules that have been identified in preceding steps. In other words, design progresses from a "global" overview of the problem, down to the precise programming tactics that must be used in order to cope with each small step of the solution. Programs are made as modular as possible: Algorithms that are used frequently are placed in subroutines that can be invoked as many times as necessary by the main program. Another distinguishing feature of structured programming is that the "logic flow" within every module is kept as simple as possible. Statements are executed in sequence from the "top," or beginning, of the program to the "bottom," or end. Whenever the logic flow must go backward (i.e., back in the direction of the beginning of the module), it is permitted to do so only through carefully designed "looping" syntax, the use of which minimizes the chance of logic errors. The logic flow in a carefully structured program resembles a river that flows from top to bottom, invoking subroutines and clearly discernible loops along the way. By contrast, in an unstructured approach the logic flow is often more like a mess of spaghetti. Structured programs are much easier to check and to verify than "spaghetti-like" programs.

Another fairly popular design technique is HIPO — *Hierarchical Input, Process, and Output.* HIPO is largely a documentation technique that emphasizes the clear, logical structuring of the processes in a program. According to a HIPO technique, a program should be represented somewhat like an "organization chart" with a hierarchy of logical subsegments. In turn, each of these segments can be expanded to demonstrate clearly the input it receives, the process it carries out, and the output it produces. The overall logic of a program thus becomes evident at a glance, and on the detailed level, the precise operation of each logical module of the program can be examined easily.

Meta stepwise refinement is a design method by which programs are broken into progressively smaller and smaller sections, subsections, and sub-subsections until the level of individual statements in a programming language is reached.

In addition to these design techniques, the development process itself can be organized to facilitate efficient programming that is as free from error as possible. In the *Chief Programmer Team* concept, the programmers assigned to a task are organized as one chief, one backup chief, a programming secretary (whose job it is to perform all the necessary paperwork and documentation to ensure that there are no misunderstandings between team members working on different parts of the project), and a number of programmers, each of whom will be assigned to do specific tasks.

Another interesting approach to the programming process makes use of the *structured walkthrough:* A programmer who designs a module of a program must justify the work in a conference to a "devil's advocate," whose job it is to find errors in that program if possible. When such meetings take place on a regular, frequent basis throughout the development cycle, logic errors may be discovered early.

Another successful technique that has been used in some places is the maintenance of a *system development library* of routines that have already been tested and proved correct. Thus, programmers working on new projects can string together these already tested routines and can thereby avoid duplicating a lot of development effort.

Documentation

Inherent in the design of any software system should be the writing of all the documentation that is required to make software a useable product as opposed to a mysterious, jury-rigged "black box." There are three levels of documentation: user documentation, program documentation, and system documentation.

User documentation permits the end users of a piece of software to employ it for the purpose for which it was intended, without reference to any other information. The users should be provided with a "cookbook" instruction manual that clearly illustrates how they are to provide input to the program and what kind of output they will receive from it. A few sample interactions between user and program will probably be included.

Program documentation, by contrast, provides all the minute details that permit a computer programmer other than the original developer to understand and, if necessary, to modify a program. The purpose of each program will be described. The acceptable range and types of input will be clearly identified, and the kinds of output that can be expected will also be specified, with examples. Each logical segment, or module, of the program will be clearly identified. For each segment, the necessary input will be documented. The logic, defined algorithms, and calculations used in each segment will be clearly specified and referenced. The output produced by each logical module will also be stated. Finally, a complete listing of the source program will be given, so that any programmer who reads this document will be able to correct or modify the program in the future.

System documentation is the final level of documentation that permits a systems analyst or a programmer/analyst to see where each program fits into the overall software environment of the computer system being used. Few programs stand alone, especially in database applications or in systems in which many commonly used routines are invoked by numerous programs that are otherwise unrelated.

This documentation should be created throughout the entire software development process. Certainly, no software development effort is complete until this essential work has been done.

THE CODING PHASE

As we have seen, the coding of a program should be a relatively trivial job, provided that an adequate design has been carried out. This part is the work that programmers love to do and that naive employers usually expect to see them doing. In fact, it should be remembered that to competent programmers who are familiar with the language that they are using, this is the easiest and least time-consuming phase of software development.

THE TESTING PHASE: EXTERMINATING BUGS

Those who have had much experience with software have usually learned the hard way that they should never trust a program that appears to be working properly. They know that a "debugged" program that has been "thoroughly" tested is simply in a quiescent phase of its existence: It is saving up one or more obscure and completely destructive programming errors to spring upon the unsuspecting user, who has been lulled into a false sense of security!

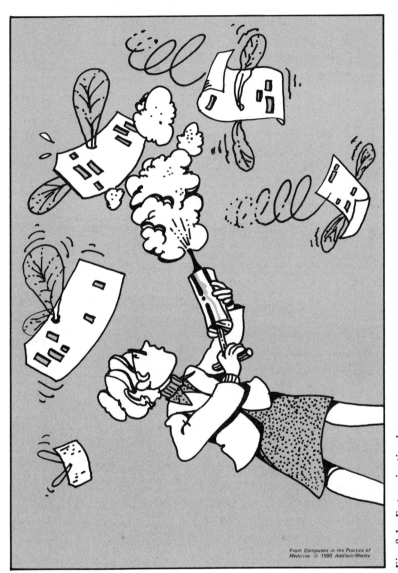

From Computers in the Practice of
Medicine. © 1980 Addison-Wesley

Fig. 3.1. Exterminating bugs in software is a never-ending job. That's one reason why software maintenance is so important. Another reason is the need to constantly improve software to meet changing requirements.

"Bugs" in programming are side effects of the software development process. Some bugs are obvious: Mistakes in the syntax of programming statements (i.e., using a command improperly) will often prevent a program from operating at all, and such errors must be corrected before any output can be produced. But the most pernicious kind of bug arises from *logical* errors in the program itself. Although every individual line of code may be syntactically correct, the effect of the programming may be erroneous — that is, it may not produce the kinds of calculations, data manipulations, or output that are required.

There can be several sources of such errors. If system analysts do not understand the nature of the problem they are attempting to solve with automation, they will not be able to design an appropriate program. However, even if they do understand the problem, they may still make errors, and the design may not solve the problem at hand. On the next step down the hierarchy, programmers may misconstrue the systems analyst's intentions. When this is the case, the programmer may create a "perfect" program — but one that misses the point entirely. On the other hand, a programmer may understand what is required but may have problems in translating specifications into the appropriate coding, and thus may inadvertently write a program other than the one intended.

Some logical bugs produced by one of these problems or a combination of them announce their presence to all by producing drastic manifestations such as garbled output. Other bugs are more subtle in their effect, but are still detectable by wary users. For instance, a programming error that produces an incorrect result in a statistical test may yield numeric values that are plausible but actually erroneous. The user who takes a computer's word for any relatively simple calculation without checking at least a few samples for accuracy is playing a risky game. We are aware of a "home brew" statistics package that had been used by physicians for over a year before anyone noticed an error in the Student's t test. Who knows how many papers with false statistical "conclusions" have been published, thanks to such programs? Reviewers rarely run checks, and they rarely have the raw data even if they wish to check it.

When a statistical software package has been widely used on a particular machine for a long period of time, most bugs will eventually be detected and corrected; users will thus have reasonable confidence in the package. But even so, users remain responsible for checking the accuracy of results. If a scientist publishes a statistical analysis that is subsequently proved to be erroneous, blaming the programmer is a rather lame excuse!

Although subtle programming errors are frustrating enough, they are unfortunately not the most obscure: They at least announce their presence, however faintly, by giving invalid results. The most occult bugs in a program may lie dormant in parts of the code that have never even been tested. How can this be?

Most of the time it is impossible to give all conceivable sets of input to a computer program. The potential variation in input may be literally infinite. At most, those testing a program with sample data usually have to settle for input at the extremes of the expected range of values, plus the few samples from within that range. Sometimes programmers will include special routines in their programs that will identify and reject input that falls outside a specified range of acceptable values. Sometimes they will even make sure that these routines function properly by throwing a few erroneous input sets at the program. But not always. After months and months of error-free execution, a program may be thrown into disastrous turmoil by a data entry clerk who makes an incorrect key stroke — for instance, putting a negative sign in front of a number where none was expected or planned for. There are many other input errors that can fool a program that works perfectly if it is given correct input.

In very general terms, we can identify four levels of program testing. The first and easiest is to submit a few sample sets of "typical" data to a program, and to verify the correctness of the results produced. At a second and slightly more rigorous level, programs can be tested with a broad set of sample input that varies at regular intervals throughout the range of possible correct input.

Neither one of these levels of testing does anything to determine what happens when a program encounters improper input. What happens, for example, if a clerk makes a typing error and gives the computer alphabetical characters when it wants numbers? Programmers should always anticipate such problems — but sometimes

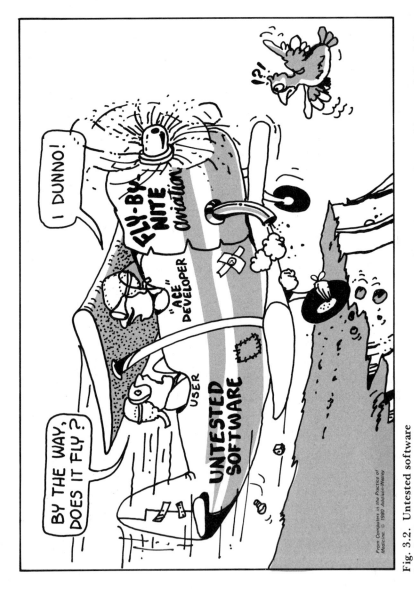

Fig. 3.2. Untested software
It is foolhardy to assume that a program works properly unless it has been thoroughly tested. Don't let yourself be "taken for a ride!"

they don't. When they do anticipate such problems, developers may include "error-detection routines" in their programs. Unfortunately, it is not uncommon for software developers to feel that they have discharged their duty by including these routines in their work, and they are not always moved to *test* them (Fig. 3.2).

The third level of software testing, therefore, throws a complete spectrum of input at the computer, including input that is out of range, or even of the wrong data type. The resulting output is scrutinized to determine whether the computer detected these mistakes. For example, a statistical program that assumes zeroes for missing data would yield patently incorrect results. When data is missing, the program must detect the fact and report it to the user.

It is seldom possible to proceed beyond this kind of program verification. The ultimate and fourth level of program testing consists of producing mathematical proofs for the logic of a program. Proof for even the simplest of routines may run into many pages of complex mathematics; embarrassingly, some simple programs that have been "proved" correct by such a method have subsequently been shown to be in error. [6] Rigorous proof for a typical large program is obviously impossible at present.

SOFTWARE MAINTENANCE

Most "completed" software, then, harbors errors. In programs of any complexity it may literally be impossible to ever eliminate all bugs. An operating system, for example, will always contain several serious errors when it is first released. The most rigorous testing by the company that supplies the software will have failed to reveal these hidden problems. Only as users subject the operating system to an enormous variety of uses will some of the bugs emerge from the woodwork. Efforts to correct bugs in systems programming may introduce new bugs of their own. *Patches* to fix the problem in an operating system may themselves have to be patched in the future. For this reason, software maintenance is a never-ending process that requires continuing monetary commitment.

Frederick P. Brooks, Jr., in his highly readable *The Mythical Man-Month: Essays on Software Engineering,* explains software maintenance thus:

> A program doesn't stop changing when it is delivered for customer use. The changes after delivery are called *program maintenance,* but the process is fundamentally different from hardware maintenance. . . . Program maintenance involves no cleaning, lubrication or repair of deterioration. It consists chiefly of changes that repair design defects. [7]

In this sense, the word "maintenance" is a misleading euphemism. Nothing is being "maintained": The word simply denotes the eventual detection and correction of errors that should not have occurred in the first place.

Software maintenance is an expensive process that Brooks estimates to be typically 40 percent or more of the cost of developing a program. As we saw, Zelkowitz thinks that this figure may be closer to 70 percent. Interestingly, the cost is influenced by the number of users: More users find more errors!

Therefore, it is wishful thinking for the user of a medical-computing system to avoid a software maintenance contract, in spite of its high cost. The user can pay the developer now or pay even more later.

So significant are the demands of software maintenance that Brooks has seriously suggested that the first version of any large software system should be thrown away, and that the whole thing should be rewritten a second time in order to correct all of the design mistakes that were incorporated in the first working version.

PROJECT MANAGEMENT

Throughout the development process, the importance of overall project management cannot be overemphasized. The necessity of close project management has been repeatedly demonstrated by software development projects that have severely overrun their schedules under the benign neglect of a management that does not know what is going on. Frequent checkpoints and demonstrable benchmarks of progress in the development of a software system are the only reliable ways of determining how close to schedule a given project may be. Function is the only reliable measurement of success. The number of lines of "completed" code that have been written means nothing. Confident assertions that a program is "90-percent complete" often have really meant that 90 percent of the effort (i.e., testing, debugging, and software maintenance) remains to be done. [8]

THE BOTTOM LINE

The current limitations of software engineering usually come as a shock to computer-naive users who might expect any product that they buy — including a computer system — to function properly. Our inability to *prove* the validity of most software comes as no surprise to programmers, but it naturally leaves users who put their money on the line with a sense of profound insecurity.

The modern programming techniques that have been developed in an effort to cope with this problem are limited and only partially successful. Furthermore, the techniques of software engineering are rather recent developments. Although these techniques are now taught in many undergraduate computer science curricula at the university level, the majority of the programmers now in the labor force have had little (if any) formal exposure to them. To make matters even worse, these modern programming methods are initially time-consuming and confining in comparison to ad lib, "unstructured" programming. In the small software development group, these techniques are often ignored in the interest of expediency, as overworked programmers try to turn out as many "functional" programs as possible in as short a time as they can. This situation often arises in a medical-computing lab. When rushed, however, programmers often tend to "design" their programs while they write them — in other words, without any advanced planning. Such haste often makes waste.

These observations have important implications for computing in the medical environment.

In the medical field it is exceptional to see the kind of design or coding of application software that would meet any criteria of good software engineering or that could pass any standard testing process. Commercial developers of medical-computer systems are seldom asked by their clients to prove that their software products have been intelligently designed, documented, or, for that matter, tested. Developers have their corporate reputations to protect and they may have large, highly trained, and highly paid staffs at their disposal. Yet they may still not be wise enough to take these matters into account.

On the other hand, it is assumed that in-house developers will naturally do their very best on behalf of their medical employers. Unfortunately, "best" is frequently interpreted — both by developers and by their medical employers — in terms of speed of generating untested, unstructured, undocumented programs. Many in-house medical-computing departments are so small and so underfunded that they cannot afford a proper program development team. Consequently, the disciplined, professional approach to programming to which the team approach commends itself is the exception and not the rule in medical-computing labs. Traditional (that is, sloppy) programming and all its attendant pitfalls are typical of what one expects to find in application software in a medical environment.

The inherent unreliability of almost all software, both at the systems level and at the applications level, means that health-care workers have a responsibility to mistrust computer output. To assume that programmers understand how to evaluate output concerning what may be to them an arcane medical subject is dangerous. For instance, a computer-generated pulmonary function report may seem acceptable to a programmer, but only a physician can reasonably be expected to evaluate the output for clinical correctness. Until a program has proved its reliability in many uses, the outputs of which have been verified, high suspicion of that program's output is mandatory. Even after extensive testing, a kernel of suspicion should remain.

Although the realities of software engineering have important implications for health-care workers who hire others to develop software for them, these realities also have an important message for computer hobbyists. A few years ago, with the prospect of the home computer "revolution" on the horizon, it was not uncommon for computer-naive physicians to assume that with a little training they could program their own computers. Anything may be possible, but the extreme complexity of good computer programming for anything except trivial tasks obviously excludes it from the realm of hobbies and crafts. The average physician has neither the time nor the training to be able to program useful medical applications. Developing a few "adding machine" routines for accounts receivable on an office microcomputer may be within the realm of feasibility for physicians who are interested in dabbling with computers: If they make mistakes, they hurt no one but themselves. On the other hand, it is highly doubtful that any dilettante programmer could ever learn enough to write the software for a coronary care monitoring system: Indeed, it would be unethical for an amateur to try out home-brew software on human guinea pigs.

That is not to say, however, that users have no part in the software engineering process. On the contrary, in small development operations a health-care worker who knows something about computer programming, if only as a hobby, can at least help to improve the quality of the programmer's work by playing "devil's advocate." Sitting down with the programmer and performing a structured walk-through of his or her program may help the programmer to see logical problems before they become buried as obscure bugs in a "completed" program.

In the planning stage, even computer-naive physicians have a vital part to play in explaining to software developers precisely what it is that they require.

The physician, hospital administrator, or other health-care worker who becomes deeply involved in medical computing will need to keep abreast of current development in the software engineering field. Fortunately, there are several avenues of continuing education that are open to such individuals.

A number of magazines are available, and some of the more useful of these are even free. No one who claims an interest in data processing can afford to be without *Datamation*. This monthly commerical magazine features excellent review articles on all aspects of data processing, frequently written by leading experts in the field. It strikes a nice balance between adequate technical detail and readability. Better still, it is frequently sent free of charge to individuals who have a legitimate business interest in data processing. Medical-computing personnel should apply directly to that magazine. Similarly, there are many other useful magazines available. Although we cannot mention all of them here, we would draw readers' attention to *Mini/Micro Systems* and *Canadian Datasystems*. There is also a host of scholarly, technical publications that data processing experts should be familiar with and that periodically have articles of interest to health-care workers searching for information about software engineering. Publications of the Association for Computing Machinery (ACM) and of the Institute of Electronics and Electrical Engineers (IEEE) are frequently interesting, and readers should direct their inquiries to these organizations for complete publications lists.

Finally, a variety of university courses and short commercial courses on software engineering intended for the business community are becoming available.

This continuing effort at self-education will obviously not transform a health-care professional into a computer scientist. However, educated consumers are more likely to get what they want than naive clients with more money than technical knowledge. Customers who appreciate the general principles of sound software engineering are the ones who are the most likely to obtain substantial results in return for their substantial investments.

NOTES

1. H. D. Covvey and N. H. McAlister, *Computers in the Practice of Medicine: Introduction to Computing Concepts.* Vol. I. Reading, Mass.: Addison-Wesley, 1980.

2. M. V. Zelkowitz, Perspectives on software engineering. *A.C.M. Computing Surveys* 10:197, 1978.

3. J. H. Lehman, How software projects are really managed. *Datamation* 25:1:118 (January) 1979.

4. F. P. Brooks, Jr., *The Mythical Man-Month: Essays on Software Engineering.* Reading, Mass.: Addison-Wesley, 1975.

5. Ibid.

6. E. F. Miller, Program testing. *Computer* 11:4:11 (April) 1978.

7. Brooks, op cit., p. 121.

8. F. S. Ingrassia, Combatting the "90% complete" syndrome. *Datamation* 24:1:171 (January) 1978.

BIBLIOGRAPHY

Myers, W., The need for software engineering. *Computer* 11:2:12 (February) 1978.

Peters, L. J., and L. L. Tripp, Comparing software design methodologies. *Datamation* 23:11:89 (November) 1977.

Wasserman, A. I., et al., Software engineering: the turning point. *Computer* 11:9:30 (September) 1978.

4

Human Engineering

Human beings and digital computers are basically incompatible. There are vast differences in the ways in which people deal with information and the methods by which computers can input it, manipulate it, and output it. In the practice of medical computing, these differences will have an important impact on the ease and success with which any given application can be realized.

In *Computers in the Practice of Medicine: Introduction to Computing Concepts,* we discussed the limitations of current hardware and software technology. To avoid excessive repetition, these points will be summarized quite briefly here. The discussion will concentrate on ways to make the best of existing limitations.

HUMANIZING TECHNOLOGY

Human output differs substantially from computer input, and vice versa. A frustrating communications barrier therefore exists between user and machine. Computers have only limited capability to be adapted toward a humanlike approach to information input and output. To make matters even more discouraging, the more humanlike the input and output, the greater its cost. In most applications there comes a point beyond which one cannot justify the added expense incurred by further adapting the computer to the user's way of doing business. Even in those rare cases in which money is no object, absolute technological limitations are eventually reached. No amount of money can yet buy a computer system that will listen to ordinary, everyday speech and that will then formulate its own programs on the basis of information that it learns in a conversation.

Human Engineering

Fortunately, with a little thought and planning it is possible for a systems developer to make the best of current technological constraints of computer systems. The systems developer can design a system so that the average user finds it fairly easy to use, in spite of the inherent awkwardness of the technology. This sort of design is called *human engineering.*

Human engineering is the rather fuzzy area that deals with the design of mechanized devices for efficient use by human beings. As such, it is really an expression of the system developer's consideration for the end-users of the system — those with whom the buck finally stops. This consideration is expressed particularly in software, in which the developers will remember that many of the people who will ultimately use their programs will not be as familiar with the programs as they themselves are. Human engineering strives to calm the user's anxiety and to dispel confusion. Software writers who strive to human engineer their products use programs almost as an extension of their own personalities in order to guide the user step by step through the execution of what may be to the user a confusing and complex process.

The personality of its programmer is quite evident in the "character" of a program. The instructions and clarifications that are output by a program should ideally reflect a polite and helpful attitude. Unfortunately, it is not uncommon for users to be confronted with computer instructions that are cryptic, ambiguous, unnecessarily "computeresque," or even downright condescending.

The users of medical-computing systems have a right to expect better treatment from the programmers whom they hire to assist them with automation.

Most users care nothing for the arcane intricacies of computer science. They care only about the quality of the service that the computer system provides for them, and this is a reasonable expectation on their part. They have spent their money for a working *product,* not for lessons in the school of computing hard knocks.

The demands of human engineering are evident in the interface between the computer and its end-users (the input and output processes) and in special user requirements such as the security of data and system reliability. Each of these areas will be examined now more fully.

The Input Process

Inputting data to a computer system is often one of the more tedious, error-prone and time-consuming aspects of a user's interaction with a computer system. Human engineering of the person/computer input interface requires consideration of both hardware and software features of the system.

There already exists in the marketplace a wide variety of input devices. With this equipment, end-users deal with a computer system in a "hands-on" mode: As such, the convenience of use and suitability to the user's purposes will largely determine the acceptability of a computer system in the user's eyes. Input devices should therefore be chosen with due regard to their functional features. They should not simply be selected by default because one is familiar with them.

The most familiar sort of input device is some variation on an ordinary typewriter keyboard. For certain kinds of data entry such as the input of textual information, a typewriterlike keyboard is often the only acceptable choice. It will therefore be a fact of life in most computing environments that data entry personnel will have to know how to type — at least in a reasonable "hunt and peck" mode.

In some medical-computing situations, however, the demand that people utilizing input devices have typing skills may severely limit the usability of a system by physicians, nurses, and other clinical or laboratory personnel who do not have clerical training. In an effort to reduce problems of this sort, special keyboard arrangements for nontypists have been developed. For instance, it is possible to buy a keyboard on which all of the letters are arranged in alphabetical order. Whether and where these kinds of keyboards are used depend on the human environment in which they must be employed.

In many circumstances, there are better input devices than keyboards. Many of these are not expensive, and they should be used whenever they are required. Why ask nontypists to answer multiple-choice questions from a typewriterlike keyboard when they could more easily point with a light pen or even with their fingers at selections on the screen of a video terminal? Such input devices are inexpensive and readily available.

When numerical data must be entered as input, there are several input devices that can reduce the drudgery. A variety of optical mark recognition forms are well suited to direct recording of numbers and of responses to multiple-choice questions on a medium that is directly readable by the computer. This technique permits those who have no typing skills to record data on computer-processable media, thereby eliminating a time-consuming and error-susceptible transcription step by a data entry clerk.

When inputting data from graphs or other continuous curves,

it is not necessary to make frequent measurements along the curve in order to determine discrete X and Y coordinates and to then type these numbers into a computer. Instead, a cursor connected directly to the computer can be traced over the length of the curve: Coordinates are determined by the computer itself and data is collected automatically, and thus a great deal of time and effort is saved. Alternatively, the actual signal itself can be digitized either directly or from a tape recording uisng an analog-to-digital converter. Such input devices could be used to input values from intracardiac pressure recordings.

When human engineering plays an appropriate role in the development of the computer system, the developer will be aware of the spectrum of devices available on the market and will select those devices that will serve the needs and skills of the end users of the system.

In an analogous fashion, programming techniques that direct the input process should also reflect the needs and sophistication of system users. In an input procedure, much potential confusion can be prevented if a computer is programmed to request individual data items interactively. It can specify in plain language the data that it is expecting, one item at a time. This technique is called prompting.

Human engineering also means that the system developer respects the varying levels of familiarity and expertise among different possible users of the system. For example, although prompting may be an essential aid to one user, it may be a repetitious, boring, and unacceptably time-consuming irritation to a more sophisticated user who has been using a program for some time and who knows what input the computer wants. Sometimes the user should have the option of selecting or suppressing prompting instructions.

Another aspect of programming flexibility should also be considered: Sometimes a computer program that guides the user through a rigid step-by-step sequence of operations may impose unreasonable constraints on the user. For example, when the computer demands a user to provide a series of answers to questions during an input sequence, it frequently is programmed to expect perfect responses to questions. In this situation, the user is given no opportunity to go backwards and to revise portions of the input if they have been entered incorrectly. The user who has made a mistake may therefore be forced to delete the entire record that has just been entered and to enter it again — this time, perfectly. Thus the first effort has been wasted and must be duplicated — perhaps because of one small mistake. Input programs should also check for obvious mistakes such as values out of range, letters entered where numbers are expected, and items too long or too short in terms of the number of characters. Thoughtful consideration of the human engineering issue involved would motivate a programmer to design software that did not require perfection of the people using a program.

When printed forms are used for data collection, these forms should be designed so that data can be recorded on them easily. They should also be organized in such a way that the keypunchers who read this information and enter it into a computer system can do so conveniently. The data should be recorded on these forms in the same order that the computer requires it as input so that the keypunchers can perform their jobs efficiently, quickly, and without missing anything. These guidelines are simply common sense.

On a more complex level, it is also advisable that the developer require the computer to perform tedious or error-prone tasks whenever possible, in order to unburden data entry personnel. Sometimes it is necessary to encode information before the computer can classify or process it. When these codes are numerous or not readily apparent (as when an arbitrary numeric coding scheme is used), people tend to have a great deal of difficulty. They become frustrated and they make mistakes, because a simple slip of the finger on the input keyboard can misencode something. It is far better if the computer itself performs any encoding, if possible; thus people can input data in a human-understandable way or at least (by using mnemonics) in a way that will make errors detectable.

The Output Process
Computer output should also reflect consideration for the people who will have to read it. Again, human engineering both of hardware and of software are important.

The physical output medium that is used is one obvious consideration. There is no reason to produce hard copy unless hard copy is necessary. Making printed output (as contrasted to video screen output) is generally slower, is definitely noisier, and requires a continuing investment in expendable paper. Economics is not the only factor at stake. When confidential information is recorded on paper, that paper has to be guarded or disposed of carefully, whereas images that have faded from a video screen tell no tales.

Other features of output are equally important. Speed, color, and quietness are considerations of human engineering that must be treated separately in any application. Nor should it be assumed that the printed word is always the best choice. Pictorial representations are often preferable to lists of numbers. In nuclear medicine, for example, multicolor images on video screens are used to strikingly demonstrate the differential uptake of various radioactive materials in organs of the body. For soft-copy (CRT display) output, the required technology is readily available and presently in use. For hard-copy output, however, nuclear medicine runs up against the current technological limits: High-quality, large, multiple-color paper output for such images presently costs a great deal. The best practical hard-copy output for these images is a color photographic technique. Human engineering might ask for something better, but that "something" does not yet exist at a price we can easily afford.

The quality of print (i.e., solid-face type versus dot-matrix) is also a human engineering consideration. For instance, when computer-produced documents are being used principally for internal archival purposes, the relatively low quality of dot-matrix print might be acceptable. On the other hand, when computer-generated documents are to be sent to patients or to physicians in other centers, one would probably wish to use letter-quality print. The developer should consider this point. The old-fashioned and barely legible upper-case-only typeface produced by many line printers is fast becoming obsolete with more modern printing developments. Serious consideration to more legible alternatives should be given as a routine aspect of human engineering the output of any computer system.

Not only hardware but also software should be designed in such a way that output is legible; that important or abnormal values are in some way highlighted; and that the overall result is pleasing and — yes — artistic. For example, there are still a few antediluvian systems in existence that would print the number "3" as "003." The information content of a one-digit integer is obscured by meaningless leading zeroes and a useless decimal point. The usual reasons for such output are lazy programming, or software that is simply old and primitive compared to that which is marketed today. If a developer presents this kind of shoddy output to a user, the user should send the developer back to the drawing board with instructions to come up with output that respects the needs of humans — not with artificial output that reflects computer constraints. [1]

Human-engineered output (or the lack of it) is also manifested in the manner in which programs handle errors during execution. Many operating systems provide a "HELP" facility for both users and programmers. Whenever the computer desires to report an error condition, the user can ask for a more detailed explanation of what has happened and what is required of him or her. This kind of human engineering makes a great deal more sense than computer systems that report only a cryptic error code and that then expect the user to go away and to look up its hidden meaning in some obscure reference manual.

Privacy and Security

The security of sensitive data entrusted to a computer system is an important aspect of the human engineering of computer systems. The systems developer has a responsibility to realize the potential harm that may come to patients if some of the data collected on the system should become widely known or if it should be irretrievably destroyed. This issue is dealt with more fully in the following chapter.

Reliability

Another important goal of human engineering is to design systems with minimum potential for frustrating their users. Bizarre or awkward input procedures and poorly designed output can certainly be quite frustrating. Nevertheless, users will forgive a system that puts them to a great deal of inconvenience as long as that system is reliable. System reliability is taken for granted: Users rightly insist that if they must make the effort to adapt themselves to a computer system, the system must be available when they need it. No other feature of human engineering elicits so little praise or so much condemnation as the reliability of computer systems. [2]

Unreliable computer systems can waste a great deal of users' time. Consider the case of an interactive time-sharing system that "crashes," destroying several hours' work for each of a dozen or more users. If failures of such a widely destructive nature occur frequently, users may get the impression that they would be better off using old manual methods. The system that has been thoughtfully designed will provide *fail-soft* routines that salvage users' work and save it at the time of system failure, so that when the system is repaired the users can be brought back on-line with little or no loss of their data.

The more an organization comes to rely on automation, the less it can afford computer *downtime*. It is costly to leave clerical personnel sitting idly because of a computer failure. While a computer is out of service, large backlogs of work may accumulate — so large that extra help at overtime rates may be needed to catch up.

In medical environments, the results of system failure could be much more serious than financial loss. Monitoring systems connected to critically ill patients must never be out of operation. Computer-driven laboratory reporting systems are relied on for timely, vital data: These systems dare not fail for more than a few minutes at the most. Short of total hardware redundancy, there is no way to guarantee that a system will have zero downtime. In absolutely critical applications such as monitoring systems, this expensive reality may have to be faced and financed. In applications such as laboratory reporting, a well-rehearsed manual backup procedure may suffice to tide you over a system failure. The necessity of maintaining adequate backup methods in critical applications is a consideration of human engineering that unfortunately receives less attention than it deserves. Some commercial laboratory reporting systems are marketed without regard to backup of any kind: Their unexpected failures have on occasion thrown a hospital's entire laboratory service into complete disarray.

Computer systems are only machines, and therefore they *will* fail sooner or later. The developer who does not think of the consequences of failure in systems designed for use in medicine fails to serve all of the requirements of the clients.

COMPUTERIZING PEOPLE

Although it is critical to design computer systems with consideration for people's requirements, it is equally important to make the best use of the human resources in an organization — not primarily to serve the computer system, but to permit people to interact with the computer as comfortably as possible.

Computers are often a highly disruptive influence in the medical environment. Those who use them first-hand will be forced to modify how they used to do their daily work manually. Such disruption will necessitate a period of user training, during which productivity will be low and levels of frustration high. The thoughtful system developer will derive useful conclusions from this situation.

First, wherever possible, the developer will bring the most "programmable" staff into the closest interaction with the computer. In the medical environment, it goes without saying that it will be easier to schedule a large amount of the clerks' time for user training than it will be to get a captive audience of physicians for the same length of time.

But the developer should strive to soften or even to negate user resentment by demonstrating that the computer returns a benefit to all users that is greater than the sacrifice they must make to use it. A secretary will probably learn to appreciate a system that helps produce the repetitious numerical data of a heart catheterization report in half the time it previously took to type the data on an ordinary typewriter. Note that even a large benefit to a third party is unlikely to win the devotion of the individual who is roused from a comfortable routine to learn new, automated techniques. Each individual user must be convinced that the computer system helps him or her personally. "Payback" is the catchword here. If the user perceives payback, the system's probability of success is improved.

BEASTS OF BURDEN

In human interactions, the sort of person who possibly irritates us the most is the petty functionary who is unfriendly, not very intelligent, and officiously insistent on scrutinizing every last inch of bureaucratic red tape at the expense of getting the job done.

In many ways, computer systems are patterned after this kind of exasperating individual. Machines are impersonal and unfriendly. They are dumb. They dogmatically enforce whatever foolish procedures they have been programmed to support. They are nearly incapable of differentiating important information from the mass of trivial data.

Worst of all, computers have become a sort of "intellectual beast of burden" [3] that some human masters falsely assume can relieve them of their responsibility to think. Periodically, there are celebrated cases in which checks for huge sums of money are erroneously paid out without anyone being aware of the problem before the event. Similarly, we know of a wretched miscreant who received several nasty notices and finally a letter from a collection agency because he would not pay a bill of $0.00! (When ultimately he was threatened with legal action, he solved the problem by mailing in a check for $0.00!)

If computers are "intellectual beasts of burden," they deserve the same respect as camels, which — as the joke has it — are horses designed by a committee. These beasts are clumsy, ill-tempered, and difficult to get work out of. However, when handled skillfully, they will perform essential services efficiently.

For the foreseeable future, it will continue to be necessary for humans to get around the built-in limitations of hardware and software technology as best they can. The time may come when health-care workers will be able to use a computer simply by discussing a problem with it. However, until science fiction becomes reality, they will have to adapt their normal way of doing business to the peevish whims of computers. Human users will continue to be forced to express themselves in ways that computers can understand. Similarly, for a long time humans will have to tolerate the sorts of output that computers are capable of providing.

For the present, the best that the users of a computer system can demand is that their systems will be intelligently human-engineered to the furthest practical extent that technology and budget allow. Before accepting any medical-computing system, users must defend their own interests by asking several critical questions: Am I getting something I can use without having to learn a whole new set of skills? Is this computer system really a human-engineered product that I, as a health-care professional, can use easily? Is it the product that I truly need? How good a product is it?

Much can be learned about the role of human engineering of technically complex consumer products by considering automobiles. Although a car is complicated and has thousands of parts, its "user interface" — that is, the way in which a driver interacts with it — is simple enough that any adult (well, almost any) can operate it properly. There are many kinds of motor vehicles, but driving one is similar to driving any other, whether you get behind the wheel of a taxi, a compact, or a limousine. Over the years, there have been many technical improvements in car design: Engines have become more powerful; the center of gravity has become lower; tires have grown wider; structural safety features have improved. However, although drivers have benefited from all these improvements, they have been insulated from any disruption of customary driving skills and habits. The environment of the driver's seat has remained relatively unchanged. When one compares cars to many other kinds of machines and considers the very low level of preventive maintenance that most cars receive, one concludes that cars are astonishingly reliable. When anything does go wrong with them, parts and servicing are readily available.

In short, the automobile is a human-engineered consumer product that, although complex, is easily operated by its end user, the driver. In the same way, medical-computing systems ought to be human-engineered so that they too are usable products, readily understood and operated by health-care professionals. Computer scientists may design and implement a system, but their presence should be no more obvious to the end user of a medical-computing system than the input of an automotive design engineer should be to the average driver.

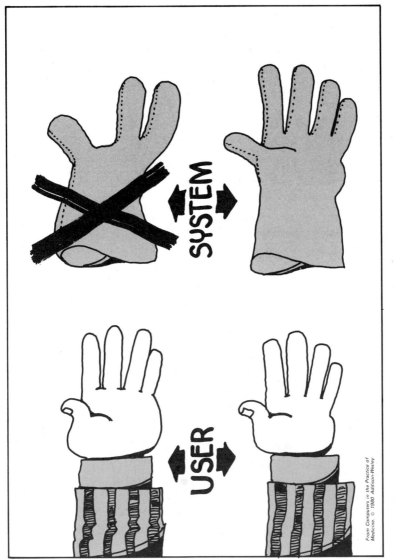

Fig. 4.1a. Human engineering
The computer system has to fit the environment.

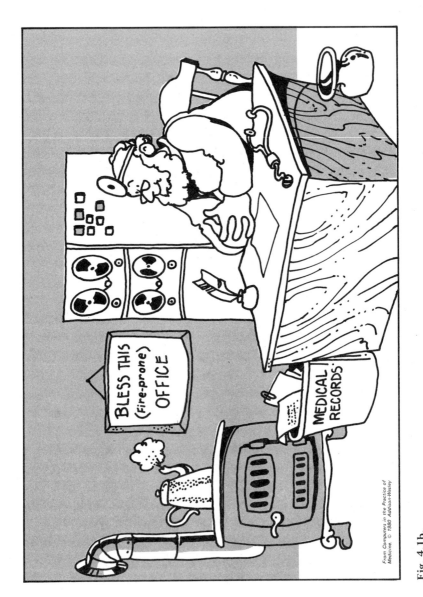

From Computers in the Practice of
Medicine. © 1980 Addison-Wesley

Fig. 4.1b.
But sometimes the environment should change, too!

In general, medical-computing systems have a long way to go before they can be favorably compared to products like automobiles. The current limitations of hardware and software technology impose real constraints on the extent to which human engineering of computer systems is even possible. When a particular medical-computing application is undertaken, a compromise is always struck between technological feasibility and the ideal system that the user would like to have if money and present-day scientific achievement were unlimited (Fig. 4.1). Throughout the life of a medical-computer application, this compromise may have to be periodically "renegotiated" as budgetary constraints, user needs, or technological advancements throw new factors into the equation.

Human engineering, as it applies to medical computing, is the humane science by which the best possible compromise is struck. Human engineering of medical-computing systems is a goal to which every developer should aspire. It is certainly an issue that all health-care professionals should consider when they decide to become the users of a medical-computing system.

NOTES

1. A. R. Feinstein, Clinical biostatistics XXXVIII: computer malpractice. *Clin. Pharm. and Therapeutics* 21:78, 1977.

2. C. A Champine, What makes a system reliable? *Datamation* 24:9:194 (September) 1978.

3. S. J. Reiser, *Medicine and the Reign of Technology*. Cambridge: Cambridge University Press, 1978, p. 225.

BIBLIOGRAPHY

Martin, J., *Design of Man–Computer Dialogues*. Englewood Cliffs, N.J.: Prentice-Hall.

Morrison, K. A., How to plan space for people and computers. *Datamation* 24:4:163 (April) 1978.

5

Privacy and Security

PRIVACY

The privacy of personal data is a problem for society to re-solve. It concerns the kinds of information about individuals that is allowable for entry and keeping in records systems of all kinds. As the IBM series *Data Security and Data Processing* (1974) notes, privacy is concerned with 1) how and what information will be collected; 2) how and by whom it will be used; and 3) how it can be reviewed, modified, and corrected.

A hermit who dwells in a cave in the woods may be able to lead a completely private existence. If he never comes into contact with government or society, he may never have to divulge anything about himself to anyone. However, as soon as some nosey do-gooder comes along and wants to put the poor fellow on welfare assistance, the hermit will then become known to some government agency.

In order to interact with society, we pay a price in terms of privacy. If we install a telephone, our name and number are normally listed in a public directory unless we literally pay to keep them private. There is a choice on that matter, but only at some cost to ourselves. If we take a job, then we will be forced to pay income tax. The data relating to our income *must* be divulged to the appropriate authority: Here we have no choice. Similarly, when we buy property, the transaction becomes a matter of public record.

Some information is inviolably private. For example, no one has the right to know your religious affiliation. However, most information — especially that relating to health care — is rarely that private.

Data about the health of individuals is in some cases very sensi-tive. Therefore, the existence of any kind of record concerning individual health poses a risk to those individuals — the risk that this confidential information will fall into unauthorized hands. At the same time, medical records are essential to the process of modern health care. Indeed, they are beneficial to the individual: Some per-sonal medical data must be collected by health insurance agencies in order to protect themselves from financial disaster in the case of illness, and from a medical point of view, health-care records can be potentially life-saving in some circumstances.

Thus there is a built-in conflict between the right of patients to privacy and the need (or even the governmental demand) for them to divulge some of this information to certain authorized agencies for their own protection and benefit.

The conflicts between the rights of individuals and the requirements of society's institutions are difficult to resolve. They are *not* subject to arbitrary resolution by data processing experts. Although such experts do have a definite role in informing the public about their perception of the problem, privacy issues must be faced and solved by society itself, expressing its collective will through government and law. Privacy is a vital issue in modern society, much greater than a mere data processing problem.

SECURITY

On the other hand, the security of data is neither a social nor a legal issue. Rather, it is a problem with which organizations must cope — a procedural matter that involves the responsibility of organizations to protect the information that they are authorized to collect from unauthorized or accidental modification, destruction, and disclosure. Privacy may be society's problem, but security is *your* problem.

The security of personal data has always been a problem for medicine. The duty of doctors to keep secret the things that they learn about patients is embodied in the ancient Oath of Hippocrates. [1] Centuries ago, court physicians kept few, if any, medical records on their influential patients, lest the records fall into the wrong hands. Even into the early twentieth century little emphasis was placed on medical records, as reflected in the sparse and clinically inadequate chartkeeping at that time, both in private practices and even in the largest North American hospitals. [2]

Times have changed. Today, medical records of various kinds are an indispensable part of the whole health-care system. Indeed, it is considered to be malpractice for a doctor to keep inadequate clinical records.

The security of these records is often poor. There are many hospitals in which anyone wearing a white lab coat can walk into the medical records department, demand any patient's chart, and get it. This situation, oddly enough, is especially true in teaching hospitals where the constant turnover of postgraduate students makes their personal recognition by the medical records staff improbable.

In the private physician's office, the situation is not much better. How many private practices are there in which receptionists entertain themselves by perusing the "confidential" medical records of their neighbors? How many private physicians' offices are proof against deliberate breaking and entering, and the theft of medical records? Often, the filing cabinets in which records are kept are not even locked at night. [3]

SECURITY OF COMPUTER-BASED MEDICAL DATA

When a computer system is used to store medical information, the security problem becomes even more significant. A computer-based "databank" can store a huge amount of sensitive information in a physically small and rapidly accessible space, thereby increasing the potential damage that could be caused by accidental or deliberate destruction or disclosure to unauthorized parties. Computer software tools actually facilitate the ease with which people can "browse" through data and link together various pieces of it, thereby gleaning information that was never intended to be inferred from the separate, unlinked data items.

Medical records are used for patient care, health insurance, costly and time-consuming research, and essential medico-legal documentation. Thus, the continuing existence and physical integrity of medical records is vitally necessary to many aspects of the health-care system.

The entire problem of security is getting more complicated by the day as medical institutions increasingly perceive computers as an economical means of storing and manipulating health-related data (in much the same way that big business now uses computers for its data). We may expect increasing problems unless adequate measures are taken to ensure the security of medical data that is kept on computers.

What can be done to guard against security problems?

The Threats

First, we must recognize the potential threats to security of computer-based data so that we can protect ourselves against them.

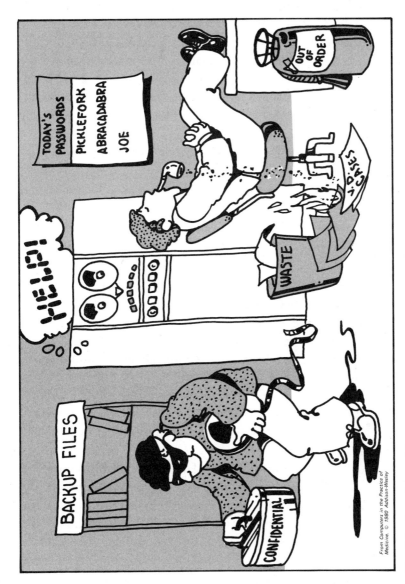

From Computers in the Practice of
Medicine. © 1980 Addison-Wesley

Fig. 5.1. Security problems
Is there anything wrong in this picture?

The IBM Corporation has outlined these threats and the methods for coping with them in an excellent series of brochures on *Data Security and Data Processing.* [4] These are the threats that IBM distinguishes:

1. *Errors and omissions.* Human fallibility has not greatly improved since Alexander Pope said that "to err is human." [5] The most frequent cause of data disasters is human blundering — for example, the programmer who accidentally erases a whole data file, or the data entry clerk who puts the wrong identification on a record so that it can never be retrieved again. Similarly, there may be an unintentional failure to perform a human role — for instance, someone may fail to record a necessary piece of data in a health-related database.

2. *Dishonesty.* More sinister human actions involve purposeful, criminal intervention by unauthorized individuals in computer-based records systems. There has been much publicity surrounding celebrated "computer frauds" in the business community, in which huge sums of money have sometimes been embezzled. [6] In medicine, computer fraud might also take place — especially where health insurance information is concerned. However, the more probable criminal threat to the security of computer-based health records concerns the unlawful disclosure of confidential health-care data to unauthorized third parties. Medical-computer installations must protect themselves against such third parties as insurance company representatives who would like to get their hands on their customers' health-care data.

3. *Vandalism.* In Ontario, Canada, a minor scandal erupted in 1978 when a newspaper broke a story that programmers in the provincial Ministry of Health were amusing themselves by collating lists of persons who had been treated for venereal disease. Computer-based medical records have to be protected against this kind of hooliganism. The story was later shown to be largely, if not completely, a fabrication. The point is that it was *possible.*

Potentially more destructive is the disgruntled employee who seeks vengeance on the boss by deliberately trying to destroy irreplaceable data. This possibility is not simply theoretical: It has sometimes happened in industry, with devastating consequences.

Also, a remote but real possibility is the random vandalism of computer installations and their data by outside persons, even by terrorists.

4. *Natural disasters.* A number of natural disasters could destroy computers and their medical data, with potential interruption of patient care, research protocols, or hospital business functions.

Fire in or near the computer room or the data library is always a tremendously worrisome danger. Fire can originate in the storage area where paper supplies are kept. Electrical fires caused by malfunctioning components in computer hardware can also occur.

The presence of smoke can damage both computer hardware and the magnetic storage media on which data are stored. Even people smoking can pose a serious threat to the integrity of magnetically stored data — not only because smoking is a fire hazard, but also because particulate smoke material gets into hardware and storage media, and can interfere with correct reading and writing of data (Fig. 5.2).

Water damage caused by fire fighting efforts, leaking roofs, and faulty plumbing can also destroy computer hardware and stored data.

The Magnitude of the Threats

Unlike conventional paper records, the records stored on a computer system are miniaturized and centralized in one small place. One disk pack may contain the equivalent of a couple of rooms full of ordinary paper medical records. Although obviously beneficial from an operational point of view, this extreme condensation of health-related data poses potentially very serious security problems.

The blundering programmer who accidentally types the wrong command on a terminal can destroy an entire data file with a single flick of the finger — a feat obviously impossible in conventional records systems. The crook who steals a magnetic tape containing health-care data may get the equivalent of a dump truck full of ordinary charts. A malicious intruder can wreak enormous havoc while doing relatively little physical damage. Fire, smoke, or water damage, even if confined to a small area, can wipe out a computer system and all the data it contains.

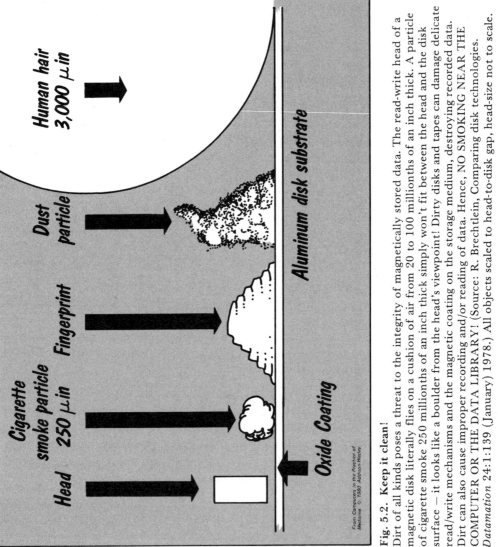

Fig. 5.2. Keep it clean!
Dirt of all kinds poses a threat to the integrity of magnetically stored data. The read-write head of a magnetic disk literally flies on a cushion of air from 20 to 100 millionths of an inch thick. A particle of cigarette smoke 250 millionths of an inch thick simply won't fit between the head and the disk surface — it looks like a boulder from the head's viewpoint! Dirty disks and tapes can damage delicate read/write mechanisms and the magnetic coating on the storage medium, destroying recorded data. Dirt can also cause improper recording and/or reading of data. Hence, NO SMOKING NEAR THE COMPUTER OR THE DATA LIBRARY! (Source: R. Brechtlein, Comparing disk technologies. *Datamation* 24:1:139 (January) 1978.) All objects scaled to head-to-disk gap, head-size not to scale.

The ability of computer systems to be programmed for easy retrieval and correlation of huge amounts of data is among the principal motivations for using them. With appropriate programming, we can discern relationships among data that were not previously apparent because of the prohibitive amount of work required to correlate and cross-index old-fashioned paper charts. Paradoxically, this very strength of computer systems is also one of their largest security liabilities: The elegant software tools designed to assist legitimate users in retrieving data and in appreciating the relationships among data can greatly facilitate the ease with which unauthorized persons can make illegal use of that data. Communications links designed to permit the rapid, authorized transfer of information between different systems can serve as a huge breach in the security dike of any computer facility. Unauthorized users who can circumvent a system's built-in security measures can rummage through data deliberately kept separate and can look for interesting interrelationships. They can make copies of data that they want without having to steal anything physical. More frighteningly, they can perpetrate these crimes over long distances, using nothing more complex than telephone links — possibly to interconnect two systems in order to extract "interesting" data relationships!

Health-care records contain some particularly sensitive data about individuals. Should such data fall into unauthorized hands, it can be put to uses that have nothing to do with health care and that are damaging to individual patients. In Canada, for example, we have heard much in recent years of the illegal use of provincial health insurance records by the federal police. Thus it has appeared that government itself may pose one of the security threats to health-related data.

Protective Measures

Considering the spectrum of security threats to medical-computing systems and the data that they contain, what protective measures should be instituted to prevent the disasters that we have discussed? Industry has responded to security needs in business data processing with a variety of countermeasures designed to prevent or limit the extent of security breaches of data processing systems.

Backup

A variety of backup procedures should be instituted against the realistic possibility that data may be inadvertently or deliberately destroyed, damaged, or modified because of any of the human or natural causes outlined above.

Duplicate copies of all important data *must* be kept. It usually suffices to perform such "system backup" at the end of every working day, so that in the event of disaster one day's work at most will be lost. A data processing installation can even improve on this by keeping a computer-maintained *transaction log* that records every interaction between users and the system. Using yesterday's backup file and today's transaction log, one can totally restore a destroyed database right up to the point where the destruction occurred.

Obviously, it is lunacy to store backup files (tapes or disks) in or even near the computer room. Although this procedure might save you from the consequences of a programmer's mistake, it cannot help you if a conflagration destroys your backup files along with the computer system. Backup materials should be housed in another part of the building, preferably in a fire-proof vault.

If a computer system is essential to the normal operation of some aspect of medical service that is being rendered to patients (for instance, a laboratory reporting system), there *must* be adequate backup for the entire system in the event that the computer is destroyed or (more probably) put out of service by a minor electrical fire or other malfunction. In many cases, the cheapest adequate solution is to have a predefined manual backup procedure to which one can resort if necessary. In other cases it may be mandatory to arrange for the processing of one's data on someone else's computer system in the event of disaster. This kind of arrangement should be negotiated *before* disaster strikes — not after!

Even relatively minor problems can terminate data processing operations, and adequate backup procedures should take these possibilities into account. A fire confined to a storage area can still destroy the entire supply of a particular kind of preprinted form, such as checks or medical records forms. There must be an emergency supply of such forms in a secure location, or one should have a good working relationship with a printer who is responsive to a customer's needs in an emergency.

Physical Security

The time is long gone when computer installations could be proudly displayed as showpieces behind glass walls. The computer room should be physically secure against intrusion at all times. In practical terms, this means a lock on the door, a security patrol, and strict limitation of access to the computer facility to authorized staff.

In large, expensive, and critical industrial data processing centers, physical security measures are elaborate and may include passcard entry to the computer room, a combination lock on the door of the computer center, or keys. Often terminals are located remotely from the main computer, and not even programmers are allowed into the computer room — only the operators are permitted there.

In most medical-computing situations the installation will be much more modest. Therefore, simple security measures will have to suffice.

Fire Protection

A sprinkler system is worse than useless. (Remember that water will damage a computer.) Fire-extinguishing gas, nontoxic to humans, is a standard fire-protection measure in computer rooms.

Fire *prevention* is equally important. Computer rooms should be kept clean, and mounds of scrap paper must not be allowed to accumulate. Books, manuals, and paper supplies are best stored elsewhere, since fire may either start among such supplies or be fuelled by them. Considering the destruction that smoke can cause, it would be desirable to keep all paper supplies far away from the computer room, rather than just next door. Perhaps the fire inspector for your institution could help you to institute a good program of fire prevention. Smoking must be prohibited in the computer room and in data libraries housing magnetic media. Naturally, all the electrical safety rules must be respected in an effort to prevent electrical fires due to overloaded power lines and other causes. Professional electricians' assistance will be required for everything except a micro-computer system that uses standard wall current.

Computer Defences

Computer systems can be programmed to defend themselves against security breaches. [7]

First, software can be designed to identify would-be users signing on to the system. Usually an account number of some kind is used for this purpose, although such items as pass cards or keys on the terminals have also been used, thus combining some aspects of physical and system security.

Second, the system might try to verify that users are who they claim to be. Verification can sometimes be accomplished through the use of passwords, known only to the authorized user. To make sure that a password remains secret, the user can change it at will. This good idea is often thwarted by lazy users: The most common passwords used on any system are probably the user's first name, the user's last name backwards, or a variation on this simple theme! Since most criminal security breaches are caused by "inside" workers, this lazy practice is a serious security problem. In more elaborate installations, hand-printing machines or voice-printing are used to verify the identity of computer system users. [8] In general, these facilities are beyond the means or the needs of the average medical-computer installation.

Third, once a verified user has been signed on to a system, the system can restrict his or her activities to those functions that the user has been duly authorized to perform. A database management system, for example, lends itself to this kind of approach: It can be programmed by the database administrator to permit specific users to have access only to those data items that they require for their work and not to the rest of the database. The database administrator can further specify whether a given user is permitted to change certain data items, add new data items, or merely view them without modifying them. With more sophisticated systems, the administrator can further state at what hours given individuals are allowed to use the system. Such measures, in addition to the physical security measures outlined, may effectively prohibit unauthorized access to the database by "inside" workers after business hours.

Fourth, the computer system can be programmed to keep a detailed record of all transactions between users and the system that notes the identity of the user, the time, and the terminal used for every action, as well as the operation performed and the data transacted. This detailed record is the *transaction log* to which we previously referred. It serves not only as a means of backup in the event of system failure, but also as a security check for the system. If a user should be informed that his or her account was last opened at a time when the user was not using the system, then the security breach can be immediately reported to the appropriate authority, and the user can change the password, preventing further incursions.

Fifth, very sensitive data can be encrypted (scrambled), both for transmission over data communications lines (to prevent wiretappers from understanding it), and for recording on magnetic storage media (so that thieves could not understand it even if they stole it or copied it). The National Bureau of Standards has developed an encryption algorithm, which it recommends for use in sensitive data processing facilities. Suffice it to say that this algorithm depends on a random numerical key that results in literally millions and millions of possible encryption mechanisms, thus making manual deciphering impossible. However, it has been pointed out by some critics that a very large computer system could be used to crack the NBS encryption procedure by "brute force" if necessary, that is, by simply trying one key after another until sensible output was produced.

Procedures

In addition to all the above measures, a medical-computing installation can institute operational procedures to limit security risks. For instance, there should be a little ritual at the end of every day in which one designated person responsible for backup must produce backup files and must take them away to another location for safekeeping. Someone must be delegated responsibility for keeping scrap paper out of the computer room; this person must throw away or destroy unclaimed printed output after a well-known and publicized interval of time. Otherwise, unclaimed output will clutter the computer area and pose a fire hazard.

To reduce the possibility of criminal intervention in a sensitive medical database (such as one concerning health-insurance information or data on potentially compromising personal details), division of responsibility among programmers may help to ensure that no single individual acting alone could seriously compromise the database. If no single person knows everything about how a system works, it is unlikely that anyone will be able to significantly interfere with its security programming without the collusion of at least one other "inside" worker. This fact has been long appreciated in industrial data processing. Even in a minicomputer-based database management system, one person should be made the Database Administrator, with the clear understanding that no one else will be allowed to alter the security parameters for the various data items.

Finally, it may be helpful to establish a clear policy regarding after-hours work in sensitive medical data processing facilities. If it is firmly understood that *nobody* is permitted to use the system at night, then this policy can be categorically stated to security personnel. In some installations, of course, this policy may be impractical.

THINKING THE UNTHINKABLE

Many computer facilities that house medical data are small, and the smaller the operation, the more likely are its proprietors to assume that a serious breach of security could not occur in their facility.

This is wishful thinking. Even though a computer system is too small or too unimportant to attract sophisticated criminals, serious breaches of security can still occur through simple carelessness. A video terminal thoughtlessly located in plain view of unauthorized personnel or the general public can display confidential health information for all to read. Hard-copy output discarded into waste baskets can be retrieved and read by anyone, including the custodial staff. Since it may be nearly impossible to prevent this kind of accidental disclosure, many medical-computing facilities use codes such as numbers or alphanumeric constructions rather than actual names to identify patients. By such stratagems, at least casual observers would not know whom they were reading information about. All of these codes, however, are easily crackable by anyone who has an interest in so doing.

Even more insidious are situations in which health-care workers themselves, even with the best intentions, inadvertently breach the trust of patients. For example, a doctor in an institution may wish to contact a number of specific kinds of colleagues' patients to solicit their participation in a research protocol. Locating appropriate potential research cases through a centralized computer facility may be a trivial problem. However, you may appreciate the negative feelings of a patient who is suddenly contacted by a physician with whom the patient has never had previous contact. What right had that physician to know anything about this patient? What right had the patient's own doctor to divulge confidential information to another physician not involved in the patient's medical care?

The ethical way to proceed in such cases would be for the patient's own doctor to contact the patient and ask permission to give the patient's name to the would-be researcher. Only if that permission were forthcoming — and preferably in writing — should the researcher feel free to contact that patient personally.

In regard to research protocols, several additional points should be kept in mind. A guiding principle should be that only as much data as is needed for research will be collected. Information greed not only wastes computer resources by needlessly filling up secondary storage media, but also is an unnecessary invasion of the patient's privacy. If possible, data collected for research purposes ought to relate to some benefit that accrues to the patient. Many patients who present themselves for medical treatment in teaching centers are under the mistaken impression that they are *required* to give certain personal information in order to receive service. This is almost a kind of implicit blackmail, and the ethical institution should make it clear to patients where the division between data required for their treatment and data required for purely academic purposes lies.

In order to arbitrate and regulate such matters, it would be desirable if all medical databases could be registered and reviewed by some organization of peers. Rules and guidelines for the use of medical data stored on computers ought to be formulated. Who has control over data? Under what circumstances, if any, may this data be divulged to parties not directly concerned with the treatment of patients to whom the data pertains? Who gets access to computer-based medical data? Where does data dissemination stop? With doctors? paramedics? research assistants? computer people? secretaries? epidemiologists? government? Does any moral consideration prevent some people who are legitimately involved in some aspects of patient care from accessing computer-based medical data?

None of these questions are easy to answer. They are privacy issues, and unlike the problems of system security, they are not the exclusive domain of the medical-computing specialist. However, medicine — indeed, society — will be forced to answer them sooner or later, if not before then after the fact, through lawsuits or other unpleasant situations.

If we may presume to offer any kind of general advice, it would be that given in the following paragraphs.

Elementary physical security precautions are effective and often inexpensive. A lock on the door and at least a CO_2 fire extinguisher in the computer room are two good investments. Bigger installations that can foot the bill should seriously consider more expensive gas fire-extinguishing systems in order to protect their investments.

Simple security procedures should be implemented. Backup of important data should be conducted daily, and backup files should be stored securely, away from the computer room.

The greatest possible use should be made of the computer's built-in software-security mechanisms, whatever they are. At the very least, each user should have a secret password that is changed frequently at random intervals.

In regard to the uses to which data may be put, any information that is traceable to individual persons (whether for medical service or for medical-research purposes) should be totally inaccessible to agencies or persons not specifically involved with the care of those patients or with the research protocols for which the data was collected and to which those patients have previously agreed. Exceptions should be made only with the explicit, informed, written consent of the patients involved.

When data is to be aggregated for statistical purposes, all personal information identifying patients should be purged from data *before* it is handed over to outsiders. It is unacceptable to rely on promises extracted from outsiders that they will not use or publish personal information. The originators of medical data are responsible for it, both legally and morally. *Security* is their responsibility, and that means keeping the personal medical data entrusted to them strictly to themselves.

It is obviously easier to make suggestions than to implement workable solutions. The idea of proposing iron-clad standards that will be universally acceptable to all computer-based medical databases in all kinds and sizes of installations is ludicrous on technical grounds alone. Computers are not "universal" machines. They are devices tailored to specific purposes in specific institutions by specific people. Certainly, the precise methods of data security that are employed must differ from place to place according to individual circumstances while still remaining ethical. For example, there is simply no physical way to make a minicomputer system as secure as a big computer system costing millions of dollars. However, despite the difficulties, security standards must be formulated and enforced in every medical-computing facility.

Those who use computers in the health-care environment dare not assume that serious and even potentially destructive breaks in security and consequent violation of the privacy of patients cannot happen in their installations. Such problems have already happened repeatedly in business, and they will increasingly happen in medicine unless measures are taken at a practical, local level to ensure the security of data entrusted to the growing number of computers used in and around health care.

NOTES

1. A. S. Lyons, and R. J. Petrucelli, *Medicine: An Illustrated History.* New York: Abrams, 1978, p. 214.

2. S. J. Reiser, *Medicine and the Reign of Technology*. Cambridge: Cambridge University Press, 1978, p. 205.

3. M. McCaffery, Confidentiality of records: an issue or a cover? *Can.Fam. Phys.* 24:301, 1978.

4. IBM Corporation, *Data Security and Data Processing*. White Plains, N.Y.: IBM Corporation, 1974, Vols. 1–6.

5. Ibid, Vol. 1, p. 7.

6. T. Whiteside, *Computer Capers: Tales of Electronic Thievery, Embezzlement and Fraud*. Scranton, Pa.: T. Y. Crowell Co., 1978.

7. E. K. Yasaki, Security is a warm package. *Datamation* 24:13:62 (December) 1978.

8. D. J. Sykes, Positive personal identification. *Datamation* 24:11:179 (November 1) 1978.

BIBLIOGRAPHY

Curran, W. J., J. D. Stearns, and H. Kaplan, Privacy, confidentiality and other legal considerations in the establishment of a centralized health-data system, *N.Engl.J.Med.* 281:241, 1969.

Ellis, A. C. It takes know-how to prevent loss of data. *Canadian Datasystems* 9:11:46 (November) 1977.

Saltzer, J. H., The protection of information in computer systems. *Proc. IEEE* 63:9:1278 (September) 1975.

U.S. Dept. Of Health, Education, and Welfare, *Records, Computers, and the Rights of Citizens*. Cambridge, Mass.: MIT Press, 1973.

6

Economics of Computing

Of all the subjects that must be considered in the field of medical automation, perhaps none is so widely and so vaguely discussed as the economics of computing. To paraphrase Winston Churchill: Never has so little been done by so many about so much. How often it is written or said that a medical-computing system is "cost-effective" or "cost-beneficial." How seldom, however, do people who use these magic words attempt to define them, and how very, very rarely do they present any evidence that would begin to support claims of cost-justification in a medical-computing system.

Without doubt, cost-justification is a vital consideration of any computer application in any aspect of health care. Now that budgetary constraints loom even more prominently, technology will increasingly be considered not only in terms of the services that it can help to render, but also in the light of its costs and any possible financial savings that it might effect. At the very least, much of our technology will soon be required to earn its keep. In such a critical climate, the advocates of medical computing should know what to speak about when they document the economics of their systems.

DEFINING OUR TERMS

Because economics is a highly technical discipline, a comprehensive survey of it would be beyond the scope of this book. Fortunately, most medical-computing applications would benefit even from a simple economic analysis. Such an analysis is within the capabilities of the medical-computing specialist.

The first major feature that distinguishes a fundamental but workmanlike economic analysis from an equal volume of hot air is the precise definition of any terms that are used. Let us therefore define three terms that are frequently the victims of wanton abuse.

Cost-Justification

Cost-justification is the process by which one elucidates the two sides of the economic equation: on one side, the cost of doing something; and on the other side, the resultant "something" that gets done in return for the investment. A cost-justification can be applied to anything — a process, a person, a piece of equipment, or some combination of all of these.

A cost-justification can be constructed from a variety of different "points of view." For example, a hospital computer to assist clinicians in making medical diagnoses may simply be a cost add-on from the hospital's point of view, but it may also be highly cost-justified from the larger point of view of society. Conversely, a computer program to identify patients for consideration for early discharge to a home-care program may save the hospital a great deal of money and may be legitimately cost-justified from the hospital's point of view. However, it may or may not be cost-justified from society's point of view, depending on the relative efficacy and costs of home care versus hospital care. Before beginning a cost-justification, it is crucial to clarify whose point of view or how many different points of view should be considered. Omitting this step is a pitfall that traps many naive and befuddled analysts. Frequently, the specification of point of view is a simple matter. The organization responsible for the project obviously represents an important point of view; the funding agency, if different from the sponsoring organization (for example, the Department or Ministry of Health), also represents a legitimate point of view. Moreover, it is often instructive to look at the project from the broad point of view of society as a whole.

Nothing can be said to be "cost-justified" unless it surpasses predefined thresholds in terms of cost-benefit and/or cost-effectiveness analysis, or unless in some other way it passes a test that permits the value received for the money invested to be evaluated. We will approach cost-justification by using the techniques of cost-benefit and cost-effectiveness analysis, and we will attempt to give each of these terms a precise and useful meaning.

Cost-Benefit

Cost refers to the dollar value of all resources used by the project. In our case, cost is the total expense associated with the acquisition of a computer system or with the use of computer resources, plus all other related noncomputer costs. *Benefit* refers to the dollar value of all resources created or freed up by the project. In our case, benefit is the total economic result — the dollar value of the resultant product — that is realized through the use of that same computer system or resource. Benefit has nothing whatsoever to do with clinical effectiveness, "benefit" to patients or to society, or anything so esoteric. It is merely the "economic" results of the project, expressed in dollars.

The concepts of "cost" and "benefit" are best explained with a simple hypothetical example based on one year, summarized in Table 6.1. Suppose that it presently requires six clerks to perform some job without any computer support. Suppose that they are working at maximum capacity in a situation in which it will soon be necessary to hire additional help. A computer system is considered as an alternative to hiring three more people.

The costs of a computer system are summarized in Table 6.1. The hardware and software has an amortized annual cost of $40,000.

Table 6.1   Cost and Benefit of A Theoretical Computer System, Based on One Year

Present manual system
    6 clerks @ $15,000 each   = $ 90,000

Proposed computer system
    Cost
    Hardware and Software   = $ 40,000
    Staff
      Programmer @ $25,000
      + 2 Clerks @ $15,000 each   = $ 55,000
                                        $ 95,000 = C

    Benefit
    Immediate Benefit
      Reduction of 4 clerks @ $15,000 each   = $ 60,000
      Billing for accounts receivable, previously written off   = $ 5,000
    Future Benefit
      Computer eliminates need to hire 3 more clerks
      @ $15,000 each   = $ 45,000
                                       $110,000 = B

Benefit/Cost = B/C
$$= \frac{\$110,000}{\$95,000}$$
$$= 1.16$$

Net Benefit = B - C
$$= \$110,000 - \$95,000$$
$$= \$15,000$$

To run the computer system for a year, one programmer and two clerks are required for a manual cost component of $55,000 per year. Note that many other potential costs (discussed below) have been assumed to be nil for the sake of simplicity. In addition to reducing the number of clerks required, the computer system enables the two remaining clerks to perform one-and-one-half times as much work as six clerks could do manually.

The financial benefit of the computer system is also shown in this table. In this simplified example, there is a reduction of four persons in the clerical staff for an annual salary saving of $60,000. In addition, we must consider that without the computer system three more clerks would have had to be hired to cope with the workload that the computer system can now handle. The salary saving of three full-time clerk equivalents ($45,000 per year) is added to the total benefit of the computer system. In this particular example, we will further suppose that the introduction of a computer system makes it possible to bill for $5000 per year of additional accounts receivable that were previously written off as too costly to collect with the old manual system. Total benefit is $110,000 per year.

Cost-benefit can be expressed either as a benefit/cost ratio or as a net benefit figure. Let

> B = the present value of all current and future benefits accruing from the project, and
>
> C = the present value of all current and future costs of the system.

Thus, the benefit/cost ratio is simply B/C and the net benefit figure is $B - C$. If the benefit/cost ratio is greater than one, or equivalently, if the net benefit is greater than zero, the project, person, or technology being evaluated is cost-beneficial. If the ratio is one, or equivalently, if the net benefit is zero, you are *financially* neither better nor worse off after introducing the new system. If the ratio is less than one (net benefit negative), the system is a financial loser.

Referring again to Table 6.1, we can compute the benefit/cost ratio of our example system. According to the above formula, it is $110,000/$95,000 = 1.16$. The net benefit of the computer system is $110,000 - $95,000 = $15,000$. .

Several potentially tricky points should be explained. First, if the organization responsible for the project is a private profit-making organization, all costs and benefits should be calculated on an "after tax" basis. Further details regarding such a case can be found in any good accounting text. [1,2] Second, "present value" is required in the calculations to account for the fact that a dollar of cost (or benefit) *now* is more valuable than a dollar of cost (or benefit) that will occur at some point in the *future*. The formula for present value calculations is

$$P = \frac{F}{(1 + r)^n}$$

where P = the present value, F = the future value, n = the number of years in the future at which the value F will occur, and r = the annual discount rate.

Third, you must define the period of time for which you will evaluate the project. This time span could be the entire duration of the project, but frequently it is simpler (and equally valid) to use one year of the project as the time unit for analysis.

Finally, it should be stressed that the mere observation that something new will break even financially is not sufficient evidence to declare that it is "cost-justified." There is no point in making the change to something new if its only justification is that it pays for itself. The benefit/cost ratio should in most cases be *greater* than one, thus indicating significant actual financial savings through the use of the new procedure (Fig. 6.1). Readers interested in further details on cost-benefit analysis should consult the sources cited in notes 3 and 4 at the end of the chapter.

Cost-Effectiveness

As with cost-benefit, *cost* here refers to the total financial commitment required to establish a new process. The cost is expressed in dollars. *Effectiveness,* on the other hand, refers to the salutary medical or societal effects of the new process. A cost-benefit analysis is expressed in quantifiable terms; cost-effectiveness is usually qualitative, subjective, or subject to disagreement. Effectiveness is often difficult to measure at all, and therefore it is inherently prone

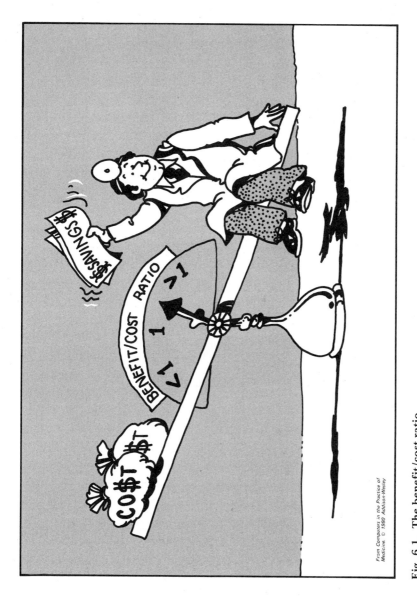

From Computers in the Practice of
Medicine. © 1980 Addison-Wesley

Fig. 6.1. The benefit/cost ratio
When economic benefits exceed total costs, a system may be justified through a cost-benefit argument
alone, and everyone's happy.

to a wide margin of error. Effectiveness can be measured (or, more frequently, optimistically estimated) by using a variety of parameters, very few of which have much scientific validity. In rare cases in which one can demonstrate a cause-and-effect relationship between a process and mortality, one has a watertight cost-effectiveness calculation: It could legitimately be stated that lives are saved at a cost of so many dollars per life. When a hard end point such as mortality is not available, then we must go to softer end points such as morbidity. When it can be proved that a certain new process reduces hospital stay or pain or that it increases the "quality of life" in some measurable way, this too may be a measure of clinical effectiveness. Of course, length of stay in hospital is a notoriously unreliable measurement of actual morbidity. However, it can be used to indicate a better *benefit*/cost picture because cost will be reduced.

Unfortunately, most claims of clinical effectiveness are not even as objective as a measurement of hospital stay. Most of the time, morbidity is evaluated in intuitive terms. It represents little more than a subjective evaluation of the severity of a disease, sometimes made by the patients themselves, but more often stated by their optimistic physicians with little or no objective basis.

The simple inability to measure morbidity in reproducible ways makes the formulation of an effectiveness/cost ratio for situations with a soft end point a treacherous problem. Even when effectiveness can be measured in terms of some parameter, it is usually difficult to prove a connection between the new process and the improved effectiveness claimed for it. Even when cause, effect, and accurate measurement can all be demonstrated (for example, in a randomized clinical trial), it still remains a thorny problem to decide just how much a day of feeling better or even a life is worth. When are we morally justified in deciding that it is too expensive to save someone? This is as much a problem for philosophers, theologians, sociologists, and ordinary citizens as it is a question for medical-computing specialists. A crystal-clear cost-effectiveness argument can raise as many moral and economic problems as it solves, especially when the cost is great and the effectiveness (in purely numerical terms) is relatively small. There are no easy answers.

For these reasons, a cost-effectiveness argument is generally used only as an adjunct to a good cost-benefit argument when one attempts to cost-justify a medical-computing system. It should be noted that if a cost-benefit argument is strong enough, a computer system can easily be justified on purely financial grounds without any consideration of cost-effectiveness. On the other hand, it may be quite difficult to prove that a computer system will have such an impact on the quality or effectiveness of medical care that financial consideration will be no object in its evaluation.

Cost, benefit, and effectiveness are normally expressed in the context of some unit of time. For example, one speaks of the cost of a computer system as being written off over a period of time in terms of so many dollars *per year*. Similarly, one speaks of a benefit of some number of dollars per year. A benefit/cost ratio is meaningful only when the time periods for benefit and cost are similar. Likewise, effectiveness/cost ratios can be assessed only when the time frame for both the numerator and the denominator is the same. Readers interested in further details of cost-effectiveness analysis may consult the source cited in note 5 at the end of the chapter.

COSTS: THINK OF EVERYTHING

It is easy enough to construct a misleading cost-justification argument: All one needs to do is to overlook some of the costs. In practice, such an omission occurs more frequently than one might hope — not so much from malevolent intentions as from simple ignorance of all the costs of a process involving a computer. It is not unusual for the computer-naive to get in over their heads financially when they invoke this expensive technology.

Such problems can be avoided when one knows what the costs will be from the very beginning of a data processing project. Then one can plan an appropriate budget. Table 6.2 lists the various kinds of expenses that can be associated with a medical-computing system. There are many such expenses. Let us look at these costs, one by one.

Hardware

Some of the costs of a computer system are obvious. Hardware is usually the first cost that comes to mind in the pricing of a

Table 6.2 Costs and Savings of Computer Systems

Costs	Savings
1. Hardware	1. Decreasing staff
2. Software	2. Increasing staff efficiency
3. Hardware maintenance	3. Reducing staff turnover
4. Software maintenance	4. Saving supplies
5. Staff	5. Collecting more money
6. Supplies	6. Decreasing use of more expensive
7. Environmental costs	methods
8. Miscellaneous	7. Discounts for hospitals and educa-
9. Inflation	tional institutions

medical-computing system. When equipment is rented or leased, the user agrees to a certain monthly payment, and the computation of the annual cost is simply the monthly figure multiplied by 12. Leasing is always more expensive than outright purchase: The lessee, who does not have enough capital to buy the equipment, effectively borrows the money from the lessor. On a 5½ year lease the interest rate generally is in the neighborhood of 2¼ percent of the list price of the capital equipment per month, although this figure is subject to variation depending on prevailing economic conditions. Generally, the 5½ year lease costs 48 percent more than the original purchase price of the equipment.

Computing the annual cost of hardware that is purchased outright is slightly more tricky than computing the annual cost of rented or leased machines. The capital outlay is amortized over a given number of years. The interest that this money could have earned *if* it had been invested is added to the annual cost of the hardware — to tell you how much the purchased hardware is costing you rather than merely how much you paid for it initially. It should be noted that the annual interest is determined on the depreciated value of a piece of equipment. An accountant's advice is required in specific cases.

When amortizing a purchase price, one can accidentally calculate unrealistically low annual costs if one inadvertently assumes that a computer system will last forever, or if one falsely believes that a user can recoup a large portion of the purchase price of hardware by selling it as a used product. Usually, the life expectancy of computer hardware is about seven years and rarely more than ten years. After that, equipment becomes old, worn, and therefore un-reliable. Maintenance will become prohibitively expensive, since (with the exception of certain popular makes) spare parts will become difficult to find and will be exceedingly costly, even if they are available. For these reasons, a seven- or ten-year-old used small computer system is worth almost nothing in resale value. The amortization period should be at least five years, but not more than eight years.

Because equipment wears out, you may have to budget over its projected lifetime for the eventual acquisition of new equipment to replace it. A certain percentage of the total capital cost of the equipment should be put aside every year in order to finance the acquisition of new hardware. This is not an additional item of cost, but it is an important budgeting reminder!

Simple rental of computer systems is rather rare for anything except the most expensive systems (e.g., hospital information systems) or very inexpensive microcomputer systems (such as those marketed for use in physicians' offices). The user agrees to rent the computer for a fixed number of months or years, during which time its owner will maintain it. At the end of that time, the computer system will be worn out or no longer useful, and the junk parts will revert to their owner. Rental payments are sometimes referred to as "silly money" by people in the data processing industry, because rental is usually far more expensive than any other means of acquiring the services of a computer system. The user simply pays out money continuously, never acquiring any equity in the system.

In a lease, however, the user generally is paying something toward eventual ownership of the system. When the lease expires, the user may have the option of either purchasing the equipment outright for a variable sum or extending the lease for a fraction of the original monthly charge. When a computer system has been leased for five years, it often has several more years of fairly trouble-free service left in it. Such an approach is therefore attractive under some circumstances.

When one can afford to buy computer equipment outright, the choice between purchase and leasing may be difficult to make. The advice of an accountant is required in considering these two options.

Hardware may be the most obvious cost in a computer system. However, it should be noted that over the lifetime of most projects, hardware accounts for less than a quarter of the total cost.

Software

Software falls into two broad categories: system software (the set of programs required to make machine resources available to the user) and applications software (programs written for particular users). System software is sometimes included in the purchase or lease price of hardware (bundled), but usually it is priced separately (unbundled).

When system software must be acquired separately from hardware, it too may be purchased outright with an initial lump sum payment, or it may also be leased. The annual cost of such software would be its purchase price amortized over a projected number of years with interest added. Sometimes the purchase price of such system software is prohibitive to smaller organizations. (Some database management systems for use on big computers cost over $100,000.) In these cases, users may have to lease software, with arrangements analogous to hardware leasing agreements.

Hardware Maintenance

With rented systems, the supplier usually takes responsibility for hardware maintenance. However, it is the purchaser or the lessee who must arrange and pay for hardware maintenance. There are three ways of handling the maintenance problem: on a contract, on a per-call basis, or with your own in-house maintenance staff.

The first and most worry-free way is to acquire a maintenance contract from the supplier. Most leases *require* that you obtain such a contract. For an annual payment that is usually between eight and ten percent of the initial hardware purchase list price, the supplier or a representative agrees to keep the hardware functioning properly, all labor and parts included. Usually it is possible to get the supplier to agree to maintain its system for several years — say five. However, at the expiration of a maintenance contract the whole situation becomes negotiable. If a particular machine has been a money-loser for its supplier, or if a machine is old and hard to maintain, the supplier may then refuse to renew a maintenance agreement when it expires. It is important to check on the company's previous behavior in this regard before committing yourself.

The second way of arranging hardware maintenance is the way most of us maintain everything in our homes: on a "per-call" basis. In this case there is no maintenance contract. Whenever the computer breaks down, the owner simply calls the supplier who then charges for labor and travel by the hour (usually with a minimum charge) and for any replacement parts required. When a machine is reliable, this procedure can be the cheapest option. It is, however, rather like gambling: As machines age, they often become very expensive to maintain on a per-call basis. An advantage of a maintenance contract is that most companies give first priority for servicing to installations with such contracts, while per-call servicing is relegated to second priority.

The third way of performing hardware maintenance is for the owner to take the do-it-yourself approach. With large and expensive computer systems that are prone to break down frequently because of their complexity, it may be economically sound to hire full-time preventive maintenance staff and to keep frequently used spare parts on site. Most medical-computer installations are much too small to merit this kind of treatment, but large ones can use this approach profitably.

The precise terms of maintenance agreements vary substantially from supplier to supplier. Parameters such as mean response time to calls for service, mean time between failures (MTBF) on the system or on its major components, mean time to repair (MTTR), availability and location of spare parts, and so on, should all be considered before signing a maintenance agreement.

Software Maintenance

The necessity of software maintenance was previously discussed. Updates, correction of errors, and revisions of systems software (operating systems, programming languages, etc.) are not normally supplied gratis except when system software maintenance is explicitly included in a software leasing agreement (and *that* may or may not be part of a hardware leasing agreement).

Software maintenance for applications programs is a separate consideration altogether. When a developer creates a medical-computing system and fulfills the terms of the user's functional specification, the resultant system should do what the user specified. In fact, the realities of human nature and communication dictate that what the user wants is only approximately expressed by the functional specification. The user may have failed to tell the developer something important; the developer may have misunderstood the user; or the user may have changed original plans over time ("only a little!") and may have thought of new things for the system to do, not realizing the programming implications of these "little" changes. [6] Because of these possibilities, it is desirable to arrange for applications program maintenance ahead of time. The user may set up a software maintenance agreement with the original developer or may retain responsibility for software maintenance if access to an in-house programming team is available. The latter approach may not be possible if the original developer retains the copyright on the software: Users who would like to take charge of program maintenance must clarify this point before buying or leasing software.

The annual cost of a systems software maintenance contract in the minicomputer marketplace generally runs to about ten percent of the original purchase price of the software. For applications programs, the cost of software maintenance can, over the life of a project, easily amount to four times the cost of software development — much of it absorbed in salary costs of an in-house programming group. It is thus an enormous expense if the software is developed and maintained at your site, and if you have no way of charging others to recover your costs.

It is easy to lie about, ignore, or bury the cost of software maintenance. In practice, most medical-computing installations seem to forget to budget for this item. Recognizing the problem and facing the cost are parts of an economic analysis.

Staff

In an in-house data processing situation, salary-related costs can be the single biggest item in the annual budget. Those who doubt the veracity of this claim are invited to peruse the job opportunities section of any newspaper. Data processing is voracious in its appetite for people, and the people command salaries that indicate demand exceeds supply. Those who like statistics can read the frequent data processing salary reviews in *Datamation*. [7]

A full in-house data processing team will consist of the manager, analysts, programmers, machine operators, data entry personnel, and sometimes even hardware technicians. Even an application that does not require in-house programming staff will still have salary costs that relate to data entry and system operation. The cost of clerical help for data entry is frequently omitted from the total costs of a small computing application! It is not at all uncommon to read claims that a computer system has reduced departmental staff requirements, but these claims may conveniently ignore that *other* staff had to be added to run the computer system or that new duties fell on staff previously unaffected — such as physicians or nurses. Such self-congratulatory reports either are dishonest or reflect self-deception. If it takes a programmer, an operator, and a data entry clerk on half-time to replace two secretaries, where is the saving? It is possible to realize savings, perhaps by reducing staff, changing staff roles, reducing management requirements, and so on. Just be sure that you document the real costs and actual savings when you create a budget.

Supplies

The input, output, and storage media used by a computer system are expensive supplies and often they are significant items in the data processing budget. Ordinary input media such as punched cards are not particularly expensive individually, but they do tend to be used in great quantity. On the other hand, specialized input media such as custom-designed, preprinted optical mark recognition forms can cost 25¢ each or more. Similarly, output media such as perforated fan-fold paper for a line printer are moderately expensive. The cost of such media increases substantially when one requires custom-designed printed documents such as paychecks or specially printed medical reporting forms. Multiple copies are very expensive compared to single-part documents. Each type of printing device requires its own kind of ribbon, which must be replaced regularly in order to produce dark, legible output. Some of these ribbons are no more expensive than a typewriter ribbon, but the big, special ribbons for some impact line printers are considerably more costly.

Magnetic storage media are another class of supplies that can be very expensive. When you acquire a disk drive, one disk pack is usually included with it. However, it is usually necessary to have at least one extra disk pack for backup purposes, and often an installation will need several interchangeable disk packs for several different applications. At minimum, a disk pack will cost $500; sophisticated disk packs that contain read heads (data modules) can cost up to $2500. Magnetic tapes, used for backup purposes or for archival storage of large amounts of data, cost about $15 each. A large number of tapes are required by many installations of even moderate size.

The employees of a medical-computing establishment will use a variety of common office supplies — everything from scratch pads to paper clips — and these items must also be included in the budget.

Environmental Costs

Another hidden cost of computer systems that usually goes unstated if not forgotten relates to the physical environment in which the computer system must be housed. Floor space is never free of charge to any organization, unless there is no other good use to which that floor space could be put. If a computer room in a hospital could have been rented to a couple of doctors for their offices, then that floor space is costing the hospital money. Even if the floor space could have been used for that much needed expansion and streamlining of the Emergency Department, the floor space is "costing" the hospital money. Two methods of calculating the "cost" of floor space are available. One is to determine the *actual* cost from the accounting records. The figure must take into account the depreciation cost of the building plus interest (calculated on a square-footage basis so it can be applied to the space in question) and charges for heat, light, building maintenance, housekeeping, etc. The other method is to determine the fair market rental value for equivalent space in the same neighborhood. Frequently, this second method is by far the easiest.

A number of modifications to the computer room beyond those that would be needed for other uses are often necessary, and their costs must be included. Special air conditioning is needed for everything except tiny microcomputers. Special electrical work is often necessary, sometimes for peculiar voltages and usually for high amperage. Electrical conduits or raised floors under which electrical cables can run are also frequent modifications that must be made for a computer room. Fire alarms, gas fire extinguishing systems, locks, and other kinds of physical security systems are expensive but necessary.

Finally, the potentially numerous communications links between a central computer and peripheral terminals will have to be installed and paid for. If telephone lines are used for communication, you will be charged for installation, the monthly use of the phone, and a device called a data access arrangement (DAA) for each line.

Miscellaneous

Lawyer's fees, printing costs for documentation, shipping bills, insurance, and many other operating expenses should come out of a miscellaneous account.

One additional factor that plagues any budget dare not be forgotten: inflation. The budget that you plan today is based on this year's dollar. By the time you actually obtain the money that you have budgeted for and get around to spending it, you may be unpleasantly surprised to discover that the purchasing power of your dollar has fallen considerably. Although this is a serious menace to good budgeting, it is less of a problem to cost-justification since costs and savings tend to inflate together.

SAVINGS: THE OTHER SIDE OF A THICK COIN

Although optimism can lead one to ignore important costs inherent in a computing system, pessimism can also cause one to neglect ways in which significant monetary savings can be achieved. The spectrum of potential savings that can be realized in a medical-computing situation will be considered here.

Reducing Staff Costs

Often cited as *the* source of savings in a computer system, staff reduction is a goal that is not always reached. The problem of claiming a clerical staff reduction while ignoring a data processing staff increase has already been noted.

In fact, staff savings can sometimes be accomplished by outright elimination of jobs. The wisdom or morality of replacing people with machines will perhaps never be determined to anyone's satisfaction, but we can use computers in this way if we so choose. An inherent problem with using computers to replace people is that all labor "slack" may be removed from the overall process. When there are no computers, existing staff can usually get by if one person is ill or on vacation. However, when a computer has reduced staffing requirements to the bare minimum, unexpected staff shortages may have to be covered by paying people to work overtime (provided that they are willing to do so), or by hiring temporary personnel. The latter procedure can be difficult because of the need for special training in the use of the system.

The effect of computer systems that are generally used in most medical-computing applications is so local that on the average it is difficult to prove any *net* saving in staff. Indeed, it is generally observed that additional people must be hired to run the computer. At the same time, existing staff are still occupied doing the same old jobs, even though the computer may enable them to do more of the same sort of thing. The reason for this situation is that most medical-computing schemes are designed to be innovative rather than to merely automate existing processes. As such, they are "add-ons" to the services rendered by the institution and therefore are new items in the institutional budget. This situation is merely a reflection of the way we choose to employ computers in health care; it does not by any means imply that computers are useless or unreasonably expensive. Far from it. Often they are the cheapest possible means of implementing some novel idea.

Increasing Efficiency

A computer system that is able to increase the efficiency of existing staff may permit an increasing volume of work to be accomplished without more people being hired. This potential benefit does not have an immediate effect: It is a future salary saving that is realized only after a period of time. As such, it is one of the greatest potential cost-saving features of any computing system. Note, however, that in order to compare *future* cost savings with *present* costs, the future cost savings must be converted to their equivalent present value by using the formula presented earlier.

Reducing Staff Turnover

Educating a new clerical person to work in the medical environment is expensive. For the first few weeks or months in a moderately specialized job, a new person will have low productivity. When a critical and somewhat complex office procedure (such as issuing reports) depends on one person, the entire medical operation can be thrown into confusion when that person quits. Therefore, anything that reduces the turnover of staff saves money, because it will reduce the necessity for employing temporary personnel or for hiring existing personnel to work overtime.

When computer systems can relieve clerical personnel of boring, tedious tasks and can free them for decision-making roles more suited to their human abilities, the systems will also increase the employees' inclination to stay in their jobs. For example, a secretary who has to type the same kind of invoice twenty or thirty times a day is likely to be frustrated. However, if a computer (even a word processing terminal) does all the repetitious work and the secretary has to provide only a few details for each invoice, the secretary can then get the job done more quickly, more accurately, and with less frustration.

Saving Supplies

Although computer storage media, printed forms, and other expendables must be included in the cost of a computer system, these costs may be partially offset by savings in the file folders, filing cabinets, and paper used in the manual system that the computer is replacing. There may be a significant saving to be realized in regard to larger projects in the area of printed forms. The computer can reduce the need for expensive forms and the staff required to handle them. Certain kinds of computer systems are also able to decrease the cost of physiological recording media such as ECG paper and the like.

Collecting More Money

It costs money to create an invoice. Someone must think of the item to be invoiced and issue the appropriate instructions. Secretaries have to type up the invoice, enter it onto the books, and mail the invoice to the client or company that has incurred the debt. Someone will have to address the envelope, put the invoice in the envelope, meter and mail the letter — or worse, deliver it if its circulation is internal. There must be some means of checking whether or not the debtor has paid the invoice, and there must be a mechanism for "reminding" delinquent accounts when payment is overdue. All of this is expensive business.

In medicine, a physician or an institution has a legitimate right to expect remuneration for services rendered. However, some of the little services performed for patients are worth so little money individually that it would be prohibitively costly to issue invoices to patients for them.

Recently, several companies have begun to market microcomputer systems for the physician's office, and larger companies have systems for hospital accounting that handle all aspects of accounts receivable. For the first time it is profitable to bill for one or two dollars and to collect on delinquent accounts. In a nonsocialized health-care environment in which physicians and hospitals are paid by patients on a fee-for-service basis, computer systems are already beginning to demonstrate the ability to save money in the overall operation of the business and to improve collection of accounts.

Decreasing Reliance on More Expensive Methods

If computer-assisted diagnosis and treatment facilities are ever perfected, it might in theory be possible for a doctor using a computer to diagnose and to treat on the basis of fewer tests than are generally used at present. The "ideal" computer support would permit a physician to use only those tests that have the greatest potential for yielding an important result. At the same time, it would enable the physician to avoid the proverbial "shotgun" approach to diagnosis in which a battery of tests is aimed in the general direction of the patient's illness.

The potential for appropriate computer systems to save money by eliminating reliance on marginally useful tests and procedures is only theoretical at this point, but it is such a great potential for monetary benefit that it merits further investigation in the future.

Discounts

Educational institutions and some health-care facilities (though not normally private physicians' offices) are eligible for a variety of discounts from the usual commercial cost of computer systems. It is a common practice for computer hardware manufacturers to grant discounts of from ten to twenty percent to educational institutions that buy their products. A medical school, for example, might benefit from this saving. In Canada, educational institutions and hospitals are normally exempt from federal sales tax and duty on computer hardware. Don't sell yourself short by neglecting to consider these possible savings if you are in a position to qualify for them.

ADDING IT UP

Optimism has a way of coloring even conservative estimates of savings. The further that one must reach into the future in order to find a potential saving, the less likely is one to ever realize that saving. Any claims of yet-to-be-realized cost reductions in a proposed computing system should be regarded with suspicion: It is easier to talk about saving money than it is to put it into the bank.

However, pessimism may make us blind to the importance of significant changes that may be required in an old process in order to fully benefit from savings that could be realized through a total commitment to automation. One may be naturally reluctant to relinquish all features of an old manual process to a computer system because the change seems to be very big and difficult. Such an attitude can rob an organization of big monetary savings that a computer could effect.

Unsubstantiated claims for cost-benefit and cost-effectiveness justification are quite prevalent in noncommercial data processing circles. In regard to cost-effectiveness, finding provable instances of computer systems' increasing any measurable parameter of the quality of health care is like looking for the proverbial needle in a stack of hens' teeth! [8] The utmost skepticism is indicated in evaluating such claims.

At this point in the evolution of medical computing, the most convincing argument for cost-justification remains a provable benefit/cost ratio that is substantially greater than one. When economic benefits only equal costs, there may be little justification for the inconvenience of changing one's way of doing business unless a demonstrable improvement in effectiveness will be experienced as well. When the monetary benefit of a computer system cannot be projected even to meet its own cost, cost-justification rests on an estimate of enhanced effectiveness relative to the unrecovered costs. Not only is enhanced clinical effectiveness through automation exceptional, but also the assessment of how much money any given amount of "effectiveness' is worth remains a matter of public policy or personal judgment as much as a question of economic analysis.

When a very large and expensive medical-computing project is contemplated — as, for example, in multi-institutional, regional, or even state-wide applications — a pilot project on a smaller scale is usually undertaken in order to assess the workability, costs, savings, and clinical value of the scheme. On the basis of such a model system, health-care workers and the people who control the purse strings can decide whether or not it is appropriate to proceed with full-scale implementation. In such potentially expensive projects, the advice of professional economists would be very useful, both for designing certain aspects of the pilot project and for analyzing its results.

The economics of computing are as much a part of the medical-computing scene as any of the other technical issues that we have discussed. Accurate forecasting of total cost and appreciation of the many ways in which computing systems can save money for their users will help health-care workers to plan for the systems that they will use and will go a long way toward guaranteeing the long-term survivability and success of their projects.

NOTES

1. R. N. Anthony, and G. A. Welsch, *Fundamentals of Management Accounting*. Homewood, Illinois: Richard D. Irwin, Inc., 1977.

2. J. G. Louderback, and G. F. Dominiak, *Managerial Accounting*. Belmont, California: Wadsworth Publishing Co., Inc., 1978.

3. Treasury Board, *Benefit-Cost Analysis Guide*. Ottawa: Supply and Services Canada, 1976.

4. H. E. Klarman, Application of cost-benefit analysis to the health services and the special case of technological innovation. *Int. J. of Health Services* 4:2:325–352, 1974.

5. H. M. Levin, Cost-effectiveness analysis in evaluation research. In *Handbook of Evaluation Research*, Vol. 2, edited by H. Guttentag and E. Struening, Beverly Hills: Sage Publications, 1975.

6. C. A. Lamb, Data processing and the user: a matter of planning. *Datamation* 24:11:169 (November 1) 1978.

7. R. A. McLaughlin, and N. Knottek, Data processing salary survey. *Datamation* 24:11:86 (November 1) 1978.

8. R. B. Friedman, Computers in clinical medicine: a critical review. *Comp. Biomed. Res.* 10:99, 1977.

7

Functional Specifications and Contracts

A functional specification is a formal description of the way in which a completed computer system is expected to perform from the point of view of its users. This chapter will detail the functions that a computer system is to perform, the kinds of input that it will accept, and the sorts of output that will be required from the system.

WHY A FUNCTIONAL SPECIFICATION?

Reality Versus Dreams

The first purpose of the functional specification is to organize the requirements of the people who think they need a computer. The writing of a functional specification gives the person or organization that is contemplating the acquisition of a computer system an initial opportunity to move vague and grandiose dreams to the restricted tableau of words on paper. It is a giant step to describe the practical reality associated with the intellectual conceptualization of the "perfect system" residing in the head of the innovator. It is easy enough to *imagine* a computer system that "reads ECGs": *Implementing* such a pipe dream is quite another matter. The selection of hardware, the performance of an economic analysis, the development of software, budgets and timetables, and the writing of maintenance and purchase contracts are inconvenient but real problems that cannot be avoided in the realization of any computer system that is to become a practical reality. When the functional specification is written, it serves as a focal point for the logical development of ideas in concrete, realistic terms. It forces us to consider contingencies that we wish we could overlook — but that we dare not forget.

Peer Review

The second purpose of a functional specification is to serve as an instrument of peer review. It forms a part of a proposal when a would-be user is seeking approval and funding for a possible medical-computing project. (The outline of the contents of a complete proposal is detailed in Chapter 12.) The written specification can be studied and challenged. Unscrupulous users who want a computer for status, for fun, or for some harebrained scheme that they know their colleagues would not sanction might well avoid putting their

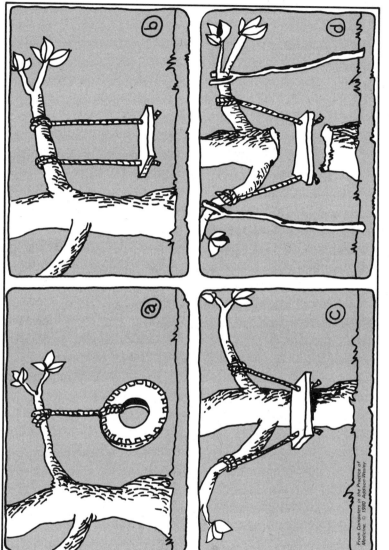

Fig. 7.1. Why a functional specification?
This user proceeded without one. (a) What the user really needed. (b) What the user *said* was needed. (c) What the developer *thought* the user said. (d) What the user finally *got* when the misunderstanding was cleared up!

From Computers in the Practice of
Medicine. © 1980 Addison-Wesley

specifications to paper. Conversely, ethical proponents of a medical-computing project will not hesitate to answer in writing the numerous questions about their proposed systems that less scrupulous people might find embarrassing. Would-be computer users who know what they want and why they want it will be able to demonstrate competence to their colleagues in the functional specification. Good work will be apparent; fraudulent or misleading activities should be exposed.

Therefore, those reviewing proposals and grant applications for medical-computing systems should always insist on a detailed functional specification as one integral part of a proposal.

Guidance to Developers

The third reason for writing a functional specification is that it is essential when you proceed to request quotations for real hardware and software from systems developers or suppliers.

People sometimes hear that computers are extremely versatile, and they therefore assume that these wondrous machines can do almost anything. But this very versatility is a problem, and it makes the functional specification a critical necessity in the realization of any computer system, medical or otherwise.

There are so many different kinds of computer hardware and such a diversity of systems software and applications packages commercially available that it is no mean feat to select the optimal system. Some hardware and some software may be nearly interchangeable, but this is the exception and not the rule. The functional specification forces the user or the user's agent to determine what is needed before going shopping. This is a good idea, since it is never wise to shop while you're hungry and since a shopping list (the functional specification) will usually save you money!

When there are several competing commercial computer systems (turnkey systems) that purport to serve the same kind of application — for example, radiology reporting systems, coronary care unit monitoring systems, and computer systems for the physician's office — a potential user will have to make a choice. In order to make a rational choice, one must know exactly what is needed before one can compare these needs to the features, strengths, and weaknesses of the existing range of products.

When there is no commercial system available to serve an application, development of a new system may be undertaken. In most cases, the user will not be competent to present the developer with an exact list of specific kinds of hardware and software. Determining the appropriate items is the developer's job. However, with an approved functional specification in hand, those who require a computer system can approach a company or a system developer with some intelligence: They will be able to tell the developer what they want their computer system to do. It is neither fair nor reasonable to present a developer with a vague request to be transported into the modern age through the magic of "computerization." To ask a systems developer to "automate our medical records" is not to stipulate a functional specification, because the set of solutions (assuming that there is a problem) is infinite. It is only too true that many computer companies love such ignorant users; they can sell them almost anything. However, the ethical medical-computer systems developer will be unwilling to do anything until the customers know why they want their new system and express these reasons in a written functional specification.

Selecting companies to approach for quotations is not a random process. By the time you have completed the whole proposal for a computer system (of which the functional specification is only one part), you should have a good idea of what companies are in the running.

When you present the functional specification to a systems developer as part of a request for a quotation or a tender, remember that you are asking someone to do a lot of work. It will require a big effort on the developer's part to read your document, understand it, and assess his or her ability to fill your needs. If you really have money and intend to spend it on a computer system, then your request deserves a considered response. On the other hand, many medical institutions and departments have acquired bad reputations in data processing circles for producing much more smoke than fire, and for requesting informal quotations on grand computing schemes that always seem to fall through at the last moment. It is not only deceptive and inconsiderate to put one or more developers to work assessing your proposal if you do not intend to follow through with a purchase from one of them; it is also self-defeating. Once a department or institution has acquired a reputation among computer vendors for "crying wolf," it will have to overcome a formidable psychological barrier before *any* of its future requests will be taken seriously. Be warned.

Contracts

When an "outside" system developer is to be hired to furnish a medical-computing system, the fourth reason for formulating a functional specification is a legal one. Ultimately, through a process of negotiation with the developer, the user's original "ideal" functional specification will be modified to conform with the very best deal available. Then it can be incorporated into a contract between the user and the system developer. The obligations of each party and the costs that have been mutually agreed upon are specified in this document and signed as a binding agreement. This contract helps users to be sure that they get what they pay for. Anybody can buy a collection of components. The onus should be on the system developer to make the hardware and software do what they are supposed to do. The functional specification serves as the contractual agreement against which the developed system can be compared. It is your only practical assurance that McAlister's Golden Rule will be followed, to wit: he who has the gold makes the rules. The precise legal requirements of a formal contract will vary from jurisdiction to jurisdiction. Legal counsel is required.

A contract in itself can guarantee very little: If it becomes necessary to resort to the letter of a contract in order to *enforce* a system developer's duties to you as a client, it is already too late. Progress can be made only in the spirit of mutual cooperation and understanding. But the ability to write a contract at all indicates that both parties do indeed understand each other and agree to the same ground rules. [1]

When your own in-house system development group is charged with creating a medical-computing system, it may be wise for you to formulate what amounts to a "pseudocontract" with them, in order to direct and enforce their agreed performance.

THE FORMAT

The format of a proper functional specification may vary somewhat, but it should incorporate sections on several topics if it is to serve its four purposes. The format suggested here is couched in general terms so that it can be used as a suitable model in a request for quotation or in a final contract. (Of course, details of equipment, software, and terms of acquisition would have been negotiated and specified before they could be used in a contract.)

I. The Introduction

The introduction will state in a nutshell what you want a computer system to do. For instance, you should say right off the bat whether you are talking about a system for physiological measurement, a system for an admitting database, or whatever. This brief introduction will start the reader thinking along appropriate lines so that he or she can piece together the details of subsequent sections into the desired overall picture. The writer should present an abstract or summary of the rest of the document in this introduction or in a separate section.

II. The External Specification

This section describes the obvious, external features of the required system, without stipulating *how* the functions are to be performed.

In viewing the computer system as a magical "black box," how do you, as the user, want it to perform? First, specify the application(s) that it is to serve. Second, describe the required input and output for each application. This description will include a generic description of the types of data involved, an estimate of the amounts of input and output to be processed per unit time (along with any peak periods), and some physical description of the input and output. For instance, it should be clear to someone reading this section whether you can accept a slow and noisy impact printer for your printed output, or whether you will require a silent, high-speed electrostatic device. General descriptions of the sorts of equipment will suffice in this section: Technicalities are considered later.

The functional specification is a document for the future as well as for the present. Difficult though it may be to anticipate future computing needs in your environment, it must be done here if it is to be done at all. It cannot be assumed that any given computer system is capable of any arbitrary modification, expansion, or for that matter, contraction. Some kinds of clinical computing systems (especially those that are essentially computer-containing instruments such as CT scanners and their ilk) tend to be monolithic and inimical to change. As the farmer said to the young man who asked for his daughter's hand in marriage, "No, sir! You'll take all of her, or nothing!"

If you anticipate that in the future you or your developer will foresee the need for additional internal memory, more secondary storage, more on-line terminals, more powerful software, etc., let the developer in on your plans at this stage, since he or she has no way of anticipating them. In the interest of giving you the least expensive system that meets your immediate functional specification, the developer's natural inclination will be to cut all frills in the proposed system and possibly to exclude *the ability for future expansion or changes*. The option of growing with your system may cost money for expansion potential in the short term, but to sacrifice this option could cost a good deal more money at some time in the future when a switch-over to an entirely different or larger system may be mandatory.

Try to give the developer a feel for the general range of capabilities that you are expecting from this system. State both the minimum acceptable level of performance and the maximum performance that could possibly be required. For example:

> This system will support no fewer than four and not more than eight interactive terminals simultaneously. It will not need to communicate with any other processors. The storage of 100,000 patient records is required and should be expandable to not more than 200,000.

This kind of information should tell a knowledgeable developer not only what you need now and what you could need in the future: It should also tell what you don't expect from the system.

III. Software Tools

The types of system software that you will require or that you may insist on being present (for instance, to ease future development) should be specified here. For example, the generic type of operating system (real-time, time-sharing, etc.) should be specified, if you know what you need. If not, sufficient detail on how you will use the system should be present so that the developer can proffer an appropriate suggestion. The types of programming languages you wish to use (e.g., FORTRAN, BASIC, etc.) must also be stated here; you should at least specify whether you want "high-level" languages and not "assembler-like" languages. Specialized software utilities such as database management systems, query languages, and report generators should also be described in this section. Don't forget to consider built-in software security features.

In other words, this part of the functional specification describes in general terms the software utilities that you require the developer to include and/or use in the final product.

IV. Hardware

At this point, a user probably will not know precisely the makes and models of hardware that will ultimately be chosen for the system. A detailed hardware picture is not essential and too much detail may overly constrain potential suppliers. However, the user should have a good idea about the general characteristics of the hardware that will be required. The more that is known, the more can be specified. To give really detailed specifications, users will generally need technical help.

The approximate type of computer — whether it is to be dedicated to a single user, shared, devoted to real-time acquisition of biological signals, or utilized by many users for database activities — should be known at this point. The approximate size of its internal memory may also be discernible and therefore specified. On the basis of the external specification, it should be possible to project the type (disk, tape, etc.) and capacity (in bytes) of secondary storage as well.

The number and characteristics of terminals, other input devices (card readers, optical mark document readers, etc.), and output devices of all kinds can also be stipulated. Performance characteristics can sometimes be specified in terms of ranges of values: For example, you may specify a line printer, the speed of which falls between 60 and 120 lines per minute. This approach leaves some leeway for manufacturers to present their wares as possible alternatives. If you specify nonnegotiable characteristics for hardware, be sure that such hardware really exists in the marketplace and that it is within your price range. Otherwise you may bias your application toward a high cost, or specify your needs beyond anybody's means to satisfy them.

V. Applications Software

It will be possible to describe in general terms the special applications software that you will need. For example, you may want to state that your software must be written in a high-level language and that a structured technique of programming should be used. You may go so far as to describe the appearance of questions and answers on a CRT screen, and you may devise a mock-up of some printed output on a typewriter. In so doing you are specifying precisely what you want programs to do. Describe the kinds of reports you must generate, the processing you need done, the files you must keep, the methods you require for entering and correcting data and for unloading old data from the system, and so on.

There remains a final point about the software provided with a system. Who owns the copyright? If the system developer owns it, will that developer's company permit you to modify the software yourself if the need arises later, or will the company insist on making such changes itself? The cost of such changes must be considered in a final contract.

VI. Documentation

Documentation standards are critical if the system is to be modified in the future. Here in the functional specification, express the kinds of literature that you will need. You will undoubtedly ask for users' manuals that will explain to computer-naive users how to use the system. However, you should also request the detailed system documentation that future programmers can use to change and debug the system. System manuals for the operating system, programming languages, and other software utilities should be demanded in this section. In addition, it would be a good idea to ask for detailed system-level documentation about the applications program(s).

VII. Schedule

The schedule commitment that you hope to contract with the developer must be finite, lest development or installation trickle on forever, but it must also be formulated with realistic knowledge of the practical limits of program development and hardware delivery. It does no good to demand the impossible, although there is considerable merit in demanding what experience has proved reasonable.

The projected dates for placing an order and for installation of the computer system on your premises must be stated. When software development is to continue in-house, a detailed schedule for various milestones in software development will have to be worked out. When dealing with an outside developer, the customer must at least specify the date for the beginning of testing, the period for parallel operation with the old manual system (if any), and the projected date for total switch-over to the automated system.

It would be wise to include in the schedule a period of user acceptance testing and a final date for accepting or rejecting the system, along with a specified acceptance procedure.

If a company wants your business badly enough, many points about the schedule will be negotiable. For instance, you might negotiate for them to earn a bonus by completing a system early. Conversely, you may be able to stipulate a financial, maintenance, or equipment penalty that they will pay you as compensation if they fall short of a firm deadline at any stage. In these kinds of arrangements it is very important to define landmarks clearly, unambiguously, and irrefutably. Such arrangements are not pie in the sky: They have previously been negotiated in real contracts.

VIII. General Terms of Acquisition

The functional specification will eventually form a part of a contractual agreement with some system developer or company. When you first present the functional specs to various companies for quotations, you will use this document to elicit from them their interest in your contract and their willingness to meet its terms.

Therefore, suggest the general kind of arrangement into which you are willing to enter. If you intend to purchase the system outright, say so. If, however, you want to lease or to rent it, state that fact and further specify the length of the lease or rental period that you want.

This is also the place to spell out how maintenance of the system will be conducted. Normally, you will want to stipulate a hardware maintenance contract and a software maintenance contract. It would be greatly to your advantage if you could find suppliers who would undertake responsibility for all aspects of the maintenance of your system, regardless of the origins of the many parts of which the system may be composed. State here that this is the kind of arrangement you are looking for.

There are numerous details about service contracts that must eventually be negotiated. For example, how long will a contract last? What response time to service requests will be the maximum acceptable? Will the final contract stipulate that spare parts be kept on the user's site? At the company's site? Or not at all?

CONCLUSIONS

The development of a functional specification is going to be a time-consuming project requiring considerable expertise in medical computing. If a medical establishment does not have access to such expertise, it will need to acquire it from a paid consultant. Trying to proceed "on the cheap" now, without benefit of a knowledgeable expert, will usually result in wasting money later.

However, those who will ultimately use a medical-computing system should be wary of seeking help from those who have a particular product to sell. Products are selected to suit the true functional specification. On the other hand, a "functional specification" that is deliberately fashioned to match a certain company's available product line is not worthy of the name. It is best to rely on independent consultants or on your personal staff, who have no axes to grind.

The functional specification has important implications for the future of the health-care workers and medical institutions that may ultimately acquire a computer system. Therefore it is a high-level management document. It reflects the opinion of those in authority and carries their sanction. All the participants in the creation of a functional specification are identified in this document so that there can be no doubt about the authority it carries. Since the written functional specification is the principal means by which developers of medical-computer systems tailor their computer solutions to the client's problem, the ability to formulate this document intelligently does not merely separate the professionals from the amateurs — it frequently determines whether a medical-computing system is an appropriate tool or a useless white elephant that creates more problems than it solves.

We have now examined how to undertake the essential prerequisite to system development: writing a formal functional specification. When this has been done, a medical-computing project is ready to move from the planning phase into the actual process of system development. Whether one entrusts system development to an outside agency or to in-house medical-computing experts, the rigorous demands of the development process necessitate adequate management if the end result of the process is to be successful. It is to these management issues that we now turn our attention.

NOTE

1. D. H. Brandon, and S. Segelstein, *Data Processing Contracts*. New York: Van Nostrand-Reinhold, 1976.

BIBLIOGRAPHY

Covvey, H. D., P. M. Olley, and E. D. Wigle, Computers in the cath lab: look before you leap. *Catheterization and Cardiovascular Diagnosis* 3:341, 1977.

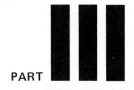

PART

MANAGEMENT ISSUES

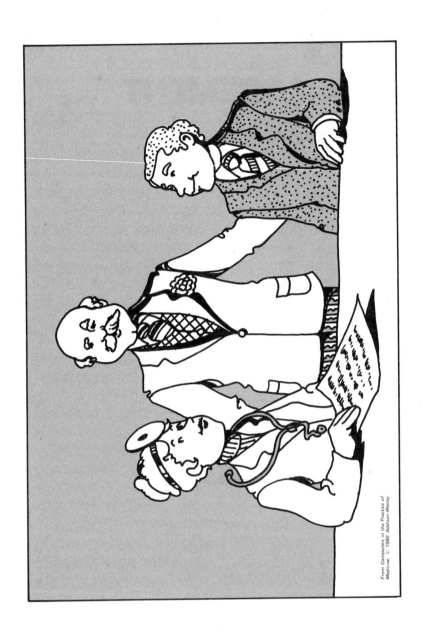

8

Managing Medical-Computing Projects

Successful applications don't just happen. The successful use of computers in solving health-care problems depends ultimately on good management, which might be defined as the coordination of various human and technical elements toward a specific end. Perhaps more than anything else, good management of the system development process will reflect an understanding of the many issues involved in this line of work. Common sense will take the manager who knows what to expect a long way.

ATTRIBUTES OF THE MEDICAL-COMPUTING MANAGER

The "common sense," business acumen, technical know-how and leadership that are the qualities of any manager are to some extent personality traits that are not common to everyone. Men and women with these innate characteristics can be trained in the skills and details of management, both by formal education in business or health administration and by specific training in medical informatics. Such people can then be honed by practical experience in their target occupation.

At present, however, the typical graduate in computer science has no training whatever in management skills, and most medical-computer installations are so small and have so little money that they tend to hire recent graduates rather than men and women of experience. Even if the opportunity to hire high-quality management personnel exists, there is often a basic failure to recognize the need for hiring them. This failure can be a recipe for disaster.

The best way of altering this predestination for failure is to prevent it by taking on a person who is properly trained in the management of computer systems development. If this recommended pathway is not possible, though, then there are some general pointers about project management that may be of use to a person thrust into a medical-computing management position without any particular background for the job. This approach might be seen as "crisis intervention." It is certainly no alternative to "prevention" (i.e., hiring a trained individual, as we shall see in Chapter 10), but it should be of some help. We will therefore look at the successive phases in the life of a medical-computing project, with special emphasis on the manager's role in each of them.

FEASIBILITY STUDY

A medical-computing application falls or flies depending on the care and completeness with which it is planned in the first place. A feasibility study should be the first step in this planning process. There are two questions that must be answered: 1) Will it work? and 2) Can we afford it?

These questions are obvious and brutal. The first important step in answering them is to define what needs to be done: There has to be a problem and automation must be potentially capable of solving it. Alternative solutions that do not require automation should be considered very seriously at this stage, since computers often (though not always) call for the greatest initial capital outlay of any method. Big financial risks are taken early in the process of automation; there is no satisfactory means of "testing the water" before getting seriously involved. If computers appear to be a necessary part of the solution, a good study will consider using existing computer systems such as university computer centers, service bureaus, or already installed in-house systems that might be shared through some arrangement with their present owners.

A person managing the feasibility study has the responsibility of considering each alternative and of explaining the implications of each in writing. If all the alternatives are proved to be impossible or uneconomical, then obtaining a new in-house computer is an option that can be conscientiously entertained.

As we have implied, economic considerations play a paramount role in a feasibility study. Precise cost estimates are naturally impossible until detailed specifications have been laid down and quotations have been obtained from suppliers. Nevertheless, a ballpark estimate will at least determine whether or not a project can potentially be paid for, either by obtaining funds from internal sources or by persuading an outside agency to foot the bill. Every researcher who depends on grants knows that there is a certain level of support beyond which a project is unlikely to be funded by any given agency. The general estimate of costs should include *everything* — hardware, software, the maintenance of both, supplies, personnel, and other miscellaneous expenses. (See Chapter 6.) Enough leeway should be left for inflation and the usual unwarranted optimism that flavors most budgets. Any other approach is self-destructive. Many a medical-computing application that might have worked has foundered on the rocks of inadequate financing — a condition that can probably be foreseen at this point even by those of us who are not oracles.

THE PROPOSAL

A feasibility study can have one of three outcomes: 1) the decision to scrap or shelve a project; 2) a recommendation to tackle the same problem in some other noncomputing way; or 3) a decision to proceed to a formal proposal for computer support, suitable for peer review and ultimately hopeful of funding. The precise contents of a proposal are described in Chapter 12.

During the peer review process, the manager's responsibility is to provide requested information, to answer questions, and to play the role of an advocate for the proposal. Often the primary responsibility for proving the value of the proposed work will fall to some other health-care worker — for instance, a physician who is applying for funding for a research project. The medical-computing manager's role is to assist clients in any way possible. The manager who anticipates objections will be in a good position to answer them: There is no better way to prepare for an advocacy in public than by being a devil's advocate in private!

Once a proposal has been approved in principle and adequate funding has been obtained, the medical-computing manager is only then in a position to approach actual implementation. Bearing the part of the proposal called the "functional specification," which we discussed in the previous chapter, the manager can now take one of several approaches. The manager may work with outside developers in the systems house, may buy the package if it exists as required, or may elect to use or to establish an in-house medical-computing group to begin the development.

DEVELOPMENT PERIOD

Whatever method of development is undertaken, the manager will wear several different hats simultaneously throughout the development process. What are these different roles?

Overseer

Until development is complete, the manager will crack a metaphoric whip to ensure that things are done and done on time. (See Fig. 8.1.) It is the manager's responsibility to make certain that the development schedule is honored and that identifiable landmarks of progress are achieved on time. In an in-house data processing group, the manager will thereby help to contain costs within budget. Even in a one-person software development "group," if it takes six months to complete a project that was scheduled for only three months, the initial labor cost estimate will be doubled. The importance of realistic scheduling and *sticking to this schedule* cannot be overemphasized. As Fred Brooks has noted, a project gets to be a year late one day at a time! [1]

When an outside developer has been contracted to create a medical-computing system, the whip is still required in most cases. The best way to guarantee that development doesn't drag on longer than anticipated is to formally specify delivery dates for documentation, hardware, and system testing in a contract, with appropriate penalty clauses for late delivery. Even little slipups should not be placidly tolerated by the customer: Remember that the squeaky wheel gets the grease!

Interpreter

Throughout development, the data processing manager will play an important role in facilitating communication between system developers and the noncomputer scientists who will ultimately use their systems. This role applies whether development is done locally or through an outside systems house.

On the one hand, the manager has an important responsibility to defend the interest of the user clients. The manager will be their watchdog, ensuring that developers do not misunderstand the specifications and that they do not try to change the specifications unilaterally. In this capacity, the data processing manager exercises "fulfillment control" over the developer to make sure that the developer does indeed meet contractual obligations. Such considerations apply even if the developer is an in-house programming team. Nothing prevents a sort of pseudocontract from being enforced even

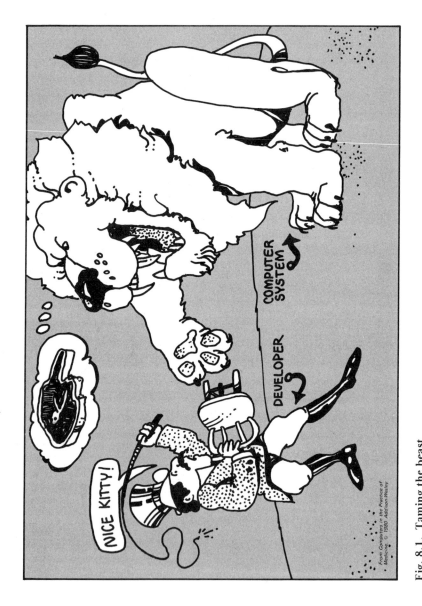

Fig. 8.1. Taming the beast
The manager of system development will crack a metaphoric whip throughout the development process.

with an in-house development group. Furthermore, economics demands it.

On the other hand, the data processing manager will also exercise "expectation control" over the users. Once a computer-naive user perceives a "dream system" becoming a reality, there seems to be a natural tendency for the user's imagination to run wild. The user may begin to attribute the yet-to-be-delivered system with all kinds of magical properties that were never even suggested in the original functional specification. If this kind of wishful thinking is allowed to continue unopposed, the user inevitably will be disappointed when the real system (that does no more than *meet* the functional specification) is delivered. Users have a notorious reputation for forgetting to stick to their guns once they have formulated a specification. The data processing manager must always remind clients that *they* (the clients) are responsible if the system developer fails to read their minds. Just like developers, users are bound in the contractual process, and they cannot quietly sneak the specification ahead unless they are willing to pay both in dollars and in postponed delivery time.

Quality Control Officer

The manager of an in-house system development team is personally responsible for ensuring that all of the issues raised in this book are adequately dealt with by subordinates. An intimate understanding of software engineering, human engineering, administrative issues, economic analysis, management, organization, and so on is essential for the person in this position, since the project will survive or die depending on how well the manager understands these problems.

The medical-computing director dealing with an outside agency that has been employed to create a medical-computing application will have to look over the shoulders of these developers in order to ensure that they are living up to stated standards of product development.

TURNKEY SYSTEMS: "IFFY" SHORTCUTS

Sometimes the development process can be considerably shortened when one or more prefabricated computer products (or turnkey systems) exist in the marketplace. When the purchase of a turnkey system from a developer is contemplated, the project manager has the responsibility for becoming familiar with each of the competing offers of various companies and for comparing the abilities of each with the client's requirements. It may be necessary at times to deliberately leave a certain amount of slack in specifications in order to allow for the fact that a preexisting computer product that may be quite satisfactory for its stated purpose may nevertheless not be *precisely* the system that you are looking for. The more exactly a system must be tailored to stated specifications, the more it will cost and the longer it will take to be developed. Consequently, "custom-tailored" systems cost more than turnkey systems. This is a fact of life.

On the other hand, it is not very probable that any arbitrary medical-computing requirement is at present exactly met by an existing commercial computer product. Exceptions to this observation may be computer-containing instruments such as coronary care monitoring units or CT scanners, in which the computer is dedicated to performing a fixed role that does not change from user to user. However, for most other kinds of medical-computing applications, the individual requirements of different users will vary enough so that at least some modification of a turnkey system will be required before it will work to any one user's complete satisfaction. Modifying an existing product is often faster and cheaper than designing a new computer system "from the ground up," but it is still a minidevelopment process, subject to all the requirements of larger system development efforts.

THE MOST IMPORTANT JOB

Project management is of paramount importance in the realization of any successful medical-computing application. It may be fair to say that professional management of system development is the feature most responsible for separating amateur dabbling from significant medical-computing work that achieves useful results.

Clearly, one person must be unequivocally in charge of the development of each medical-computing application. Certainly, committees of users have their function — but it is to arrive at a consensus and, with the assistance of the data processing manager, to discern needs, to investigate possible solutions, and to review the state of their budget. Intelligent decisions in data processing are not made by panels of dilettantes, however. Those users who do not know what they are doing in the computer marketplace are easy prey for less-than-scrupulous developers or for developers who do not truly understand the requirements of medical computing. The medical-computing manager is the one person who speaks the language of both the users and the system developers. Such a person is the only reasonable hope that medical-computing users have for getting their requirements satisfactorily met within a reasonable time-frame and within a budget that they can afford.

The need for competent management is not restricted to the system development process. Someone will have to assume continuing responsibility for the day-to-day operation of every medical-computing facility, and someone will have to be in charge of the never-ending process of software maintenance and of responding to changing computing needs in the health-care environment.

Nor is management an issue confined to individual applications or installations. Within institutions such as hospitals there may be many computing projects in many different stages of their life cycle being carried out for radically different purposes in different departments. The division of management responsibility for health-related computing on a divisional, departmental, or institutional basis can be problematic, but it must be faced.

The next chapter, therefore, looks at these issues.

NOTE

1. F. P. Brooks, *The Mythical Man-Month: Essays on Software Engineering.* Reading, Mass.: Addison-Wesley, 1975, pp. 154ff.

9

Organizing for Automation

The acquisition of data processing technology implies a substantial commitment on the part of the user. The degree to which users are willing to reorganize their approach to doing business (medical or other) will in large measure determine the ultimate success of their computing ventures. In the medical environment, there is an understandable queasiness associated with making a wholehearted commitment if it implies that the medical milieu itself may be affected by the change.

What are some of the major factors that might give us pause?

First, the acquisition of computer hardware is a big decision because it involves a large financial outlay — often "cash on the barrelhead." Once hardware is obtained, the user is locked into it. Even with a lease, one cannot simply unilaterally divest oneself of a computer, and one can usually resell purchased hardware only at a loss. The original decision to acquire hardware must therefore be one that the user is prepared to live with for at least several years in order to justify the investment.

Even when a computer user seeks to minimize financial commitment by renting a system or paying for services on a system that is shared with other users, the monetary outlay is far from trivial. As any knowledgeable computer user knows, any shared system also has unique drawbacks: The overall performance, as far as any one user is concerned, can be significantly lower than that of a dedicated system.

Another hardware-related reason that accounts for reluctance in committing oneself to automation is the realistic worry that an already expensive "starter" system will grow and thereby become even more expensive. The predilection of computer hardware for seemingly spontaneous generation is one of its more notorious and less desirable characteristics. It is the wise user who fears this phenomenon.

The informed user may become even more hesitant to embark on the stormy seas of automation after realizing that software development can be, if anything, a more expensive proposition than hardware acquisition. Rarely in medical computing can one buy a complete software package that specifically suits one's application. More often, software development will be undertaken.

Only with great care can software development costs be kept under control, because they tend to build up little by little.

Even when software development proceeds successfully, all programming triumphs are soon taken for granted, and users start clamoring for more sophisticated software. Like potato chips or peanuts, a little software often tastes like more!

When software development does *not* proceed according to plan, there is a greater danger. Because of the investment already made in hardware acquisition and software development, there is a natural tendency for desperate users to throw good money after bad in an effort to "force" system development to completion. When projects bog down and fall behind schedule, more programming staff may be hired. Far from having a salutary effect, this action may serve only to further complicate the programming effort and to put a project even further behind schedule than it would have been without additional "help," as we saw in the chapter on software engineering. [1] Thus go the best-laid plans of mice and men.

The ultimate fear in regard to the commitment to computer systems is that the first system one acquires may not be the proper system to do the intended job. The financial loss in such cases can be devastating.

Since there are numerous potholes on the road to successful medical computing, what can you do to avoid them? Obviously, timid dabbling in automation is no answer, for that will certainly fail to produce anything of value. In fact, anything less than a major commitment to automation will just about guarantee failure. Knowing this, you must be fully aware of the implications of such commitment and must organize the environment in which the computer will be used in a way that can maximize your chances of survival when you knowingly stand between a rock and a hard place! Organizing for automation should be an important prerequisite to the installation of a computer system in any medical environment, but usually this fact is perceived only in retrospect after a policy of ad hoc management has failed to achieve the desired results.

We can, however, learn from the mistakes of our predecessors and steel ourselves for the battle.

THE IMPACT OF COMPUTER SYSTEMS

Metaphorically speaking, a computer can have the same effect on an unprepared environment as does spicy food on an unaccustomed stomach: The results can be catastrophic! Let us be prepared.

To start, let's face the fact that the computer will often force the user to redefine ways of doing business. The procedures necessary for collecting data and entering it into the computer system will usually represent a significant departure from procedures used prior to automation. Indeed when an automated process is introduced for which there was no manual predecessor, medical pesonnel may find themselves required to fill out data collection forms or to use terminals at virtually every step of their activities. Under these circumstances, it is natural for personnel to become irritated at having to collect data for research purposes and to focus that irritation on the computer as the source of the added burden. For example, a computer-based data management system may tyrannically demand certain kinds of data from doctors before it will issue reports that they require for hospital records. This kind of procedure is often mandatory if complete, reliable data is to be collected at all. Still, it is a type of blackmail, and doctors may resent it as such.

The impact of automation is not limited to its effect on end users. Staffing requirements in an organization (in the hospital as a whole, in a service area, or in a department) will be altered, sometimes drastically. New job roles such as analyst, programmer, and operator may be defined. Data processing people may become part of the medical environment for the purposes of program development, and someone will certainly be required to supervise and maintain a computer system, once it is working. Secretaries may find themselves redefined as data entry personnel when a computer system takes over some of their clerical duties.

The economic impact of a computer system is usually sizable. Even if hardware is relatively cheap, software development costs are generally high, and they have nowhere to go but up. A lot of money will be tied up in a computer system — money that is not going to be available for other purposes.

Thus computers have enormous potential to *disrupt* any environment in which they are employed.

Not only does the computer determine in many cases how business will be conducted: It also may establish a precedent that succeeding generations of users will be forced to follow in future years. A functioning computer system that has finally been perfected at great expense and with great effort is not lightly modified or discarded. Thus, whenever a computer is used for some ongoing purpose, there is danger that it will actually limit innovation and change. Ideas that do not conform to an automated approach may be discarded out of hand, their merit ignored. Technology begets technology. Each step along the road to automation makes it increasingly difficult for an organization to return to the methods that were used before there were computers. Once the automation revolution has overthrown the old order of manual methods, it will be difficult to overthrow the powerful, new dynasty that has been established.

EVOLUTION VERSUS REVOLUTION

The cataclysmic approach to change may be effective in sweeping away something that does not work, but it does nothing to recover the time, effort, and money that may be wasted if the change fails to produce the desired effects. A more rational approach to a change as major as the introduction of automation is to proceed in an orderly, stepwise, conscious, and prepared fashion that lends itself to adjustments in direction as they become necessary.

Since the way an institution functions is affected by data processing activities, businesses are now beginning to include data processing personnel in the upper management team. The Vice President of Data Processing is a newcomer to managerial ranks, whose arrival signifies that buisnesses are beginning to appreciate the overwhelming importance of data processing in their everyday activities. In part, the inclusion of the chief of data processing in management is an effort to keep the dog in charge of tail-wagging; on the other hand, it is a recognition that data processing is a big tail.

Within medical institutions, the data processing picture is usually not so clear-cut as it is in a business situation. Three kinds of unrelated activity involving computers may exist in a hospital: ordinary business computing; computer service relating to patient care; and computing for medical research purposes. Despite areas of overlap, the three spheres of medical computing are mostly independent. (See Fig. 9.1.) Organizing the management of data processing in the medical environment is therefore somewhat more complex than in most industries, where there is only one data processing department. It would be helpful, therefore, to look more closely at the organization of data processing activities within a hospital environment.

THE POLITICS OF COMPUTING

Because so many aspects of an organization's activities are dependent on data processing, it follows that those who control data processing are in a position of considerable power within that organization. The fact that such power can be used in both productive and counterproductive ways makes possible a convincing case for both those who favor a centralized approach to medical computing and those who favor the opposite — a decentralized approach.

In support of the establishment of a "Computer Center" in medical institutions where computers are used, one can cite several theoretical advantages. Such an approach makes it theoretically easier to coordinate the computing needs of the whole organization. Central control over medical automation facilitates peer review of proposed projects. Such projects can be assessed by disinterested individuals for feasibility, necessity, and affordability. On this basis, institution-wide computing priorities may be established. In general, a central computer facility can possess bigger, more expensive, and more powerful hardware and software than could each of several smaller installations (this is often referred to as the "economy of scale"). Furthermore, a central facility will be more likely to attract highly competent people to the data processing effort than any one small application could either attract or afford. When smaller applications can reasonably share the same equipment and personnel, it makes sense for them to join forces to produce a whole that would be greater than the sum of separate parts. Centralization of the computing effort also creates an environment that can permit continuous performance monitoring of various projects. It can be determined by a central authority when development should be terminated because

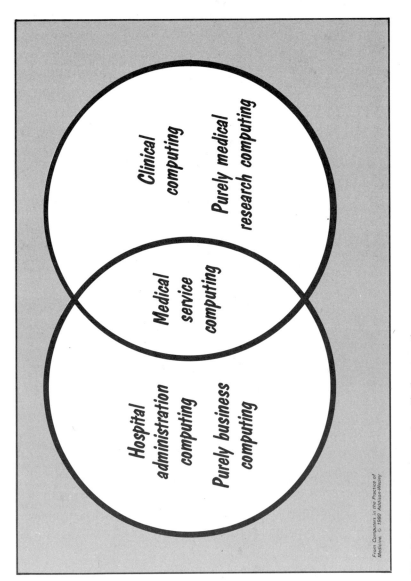

From Computers in the Practice of Medicine. © 1980 Addison-Wesley

Fig. 9.1. The three areas of medical computing
Medical research computing and hospital business computing are completely separate. In medical service applications designed for patient care, they overlap — creating a third area with unique management considerations.

of final success or, alternatively, dismal failure. In this way an institution can avoid squandering money on projects that have no reasonable hope of future success. Applications that ought to be continued can be reevaluated periodically, and their priorities in an institution's overall medical-computing scheme may be changed as various landmarks of progress or unexpected problems arise.

Up to this point, the case for the Medical Computing Center sounds irresistible. However, this approach is not without serious drawbacks. A single Computer Center in any institution can become the focus of a power struggle among individuals or departments with totally unrelated or even conflicting interests. Computers are a natural place for the power-hungry to start nibbling. A person with limited technical know-how but big ambition can easily hire the technical expertise necessary to run a Computer Center. Thus, controlling computers can provide a fairly easy pathway to a powerful management position. The Computer Center will determine what projects can and cannot be done in an institution. The manager who is not equally responsible to all interests will be at liberty to assign a high priority to pet projects and to give lower priority to rival projects. A sly fox in charge of medical computing can wreak havoc in a hen house of computer-naive users: It is easy enough to simply tell an unwanted user that a project is not feasible. Naive users will not know when they are being bamboozled.

The tripartite nature of medical-computing projects makes the approach of the single Computer Center unreasonable for most medical environments. Administration, medical service, and medical research are spheres of interest that must be adequately separated if medical-computing efforts are not to become bogged down in managerial conflicts and overlapping responsibilities.

Administrative Versus Medical Computing

First, there must be a clear division between medical computing and the ordinary kinds of data processing activities found in most big businesses, including hospitals. Obviously, nonadministrative medical staff should not have advisory powers over administrative computing functions relating to the everyday business of the hospital. Payroll, accounts receivable and payable, housekeeping schedules and the like lie squarely in the sphere of hospital administration and must not be subject to outside interference.

Similarly, physicians or basic scientists who obtain their research funding from outside agencies must have academic freedom to determine the nature of their own research and the methods they employ. Their research should be subject only to the normal processes of peer review and not to the interference of hospital administration.

However, the distinction between medical science and hospital administration becomes somewhat more blurred in medical-computing activities that are conducted for purposes of patient care. An uneasy symbiosis has always existed between medical interest in up-to-date technology and the administrative realities of controlling the hospital budget. Medical automation is making available certain kinds of patient care that were not previously available, and as such, it threatens to upset the balance that has been struck. A CT body scanner *may* improve the quality of medical care, but it is tremendously expensive to obtain and operate. [2] In such areas, administration and even government must have input to the management of a medical-computing function.

Medical Service Versus Medical Research
It is equally important to distinguish and separate the commitments to medical service and medical research. These areas are both important, and therefore clear priorities need to be established for each separately and they must be prevented from interfering with each other. Funding, responsibilities, and accountability will be different for each area.

In many ways, these two areas are in conflict with each other. For example, research projects have a natural tendency to expand in scope and in number. Unless limitations are placed on the research load, burgeoning research applications may slowly squeeze out ordinary service functions in a shared computer facility. Budgeting for both functions together is a real and expensive problem. The potential for research applications to expand should interest those who administer funds for research purposes. Furthermore, a project that begins with a research grant sometimes continues after the expiration of that grant, if it is aided by service funding from the institution itself. An automated procedure that is initially the object of experiment may be proved valuable or essential and brought into routine service on an everyday basis. At this point, hospital administration becomes interested, further complicating the issue.

On the other hand, those who wish to acquire a computer system in order to serve specific service goals should realize that growth and improvement in health-care delivery and administration occur through research. Without medical research, the theory of the four humors would still represent the ultimate understanding in human physiology! In medical computing, progress is not going to be realized by the mere implementation of commercially available systems.

A reasonable balance between service and research is the foundation on which computing can best serve the health-care community. It is incumbent on those who administer medical-computing systems to insure peaceful coexistence and helpful cooperation between these two fields of medical-computing interest, and yet to insure their total independence and autonomy.

AVOIDING CONFLICTS

In the spirit of preventive medicine, the best way to deal with the headaches that can be caused by overlapping management is to organize for automation in such a way that management conflicts are avoided in the first place.

Management's Role

A practical solution is to recognize the fundamental differences between the requirements of research versus those of hospital business computing, and to separate the management of each so that they do not step on each other's toes (Fig. 9.2).

With hospital business data processing, the overriding necessity is for stability, reliability, security, and fiscal responsibility within the institution. The evolution of data processing here is slow and deliberate, since mistakes are extremely costly and could have potentially disastrous consequences for the institution. Computer applications for business functions in a hospital will develop as the

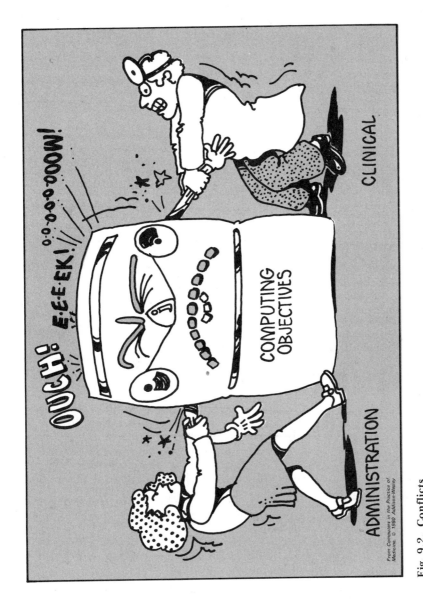

Fig. 9.2. Conflicts
The very different goals of hospital business computing and medical research computing can lead to rivalry if management responsibilities are not clearly divided.

result of numerous conferences, deliberations, and meetings. When so much is at stake, domination by computer enthusiasts cannot be allowed. Full institutional backing is required before any change can be made.

However, in computing for medical research exactly the opposite requirements exist. Much of clinical research depends on insights and inspirations of single individuals or small groups of colleagues. The funding process normally grants money to individual researchers for the specific purposes of achieving their own particular aims. Computing requirements for medical research projects are in a constant state of upheaval and modification: Those who wait for stabilization or a consensus will wait forever, miss their opportunities, and achieve nothing. The success of any given medical research project is never guaranteed at the outset, nor can it be essential to the life of an institution. Many medical research ventures have served a useful purpose by identifying a blind alley so that others will not have to repeat the same mistakes. Therefore, computing requirements in medical research should be geared to the small, incisive, leading edge of investigation — not to the safe, predictable requirements so necessary for the stability of hospital business.

Recognizing the vast differences between hospital business data processing and the innovative requirements of medical research computing, management should be separated into a Department of Administrative Data Processing for the large, central data processing functions of running the hospital, and a separate administration for Clinical Computing. These spheres of influence will have no areas of mutual responsibility except in those cases in which they agree that their jurisdictions clearly overlap. An excellent arbitrator of questions of responsibility in given applications is the person in charge of funding. Research funds support research computing. The hospital budget supports hospital business computing.

On the management level, the department in charge of hospital business computing is the same as the data processing department in any other kind of business. Its head may be a Vice President within the hospital administration, though in most institutions this person carries some other less important title, such as Director.

On the other hand, the person who heads Clinical Computing will have functions unique to the medical-computing environment. What, precisely, does the Director of Clinical Computing do?

This person will exert a leadership function among researchers and health-care innovators within an institution, will motivate and "sell" users on the advantages of automation when there is reason to believe that such advantages exist, will coordinate the development of shared resources, and will move projects from the planning stages through to completion. The Director of Clinical Computing will be a source of expertise, a person who possesses knowledge about the myriad details that must be attended to in order to implement medical-computer applications and keep them running smoothly. This individual will assess the feasibility of user requests, establish reasonable schedules, and be concerned with the financial realities of running computer services. Because of a unique expertise, the Director may often be called on to assist medical personnel in preparing their grant applications for research projects that will require expenditures for data processing.

In short, this is also a management position of high responsibility. It should *never* be viewed as a consultative role. Unless there is one person in charge of this area, it will be directionless, and no user will be served particularly well. The Director must be independent, having no special obligations to any one user or clique of users, since he or she is responsible for all clinical computing endeavors within his or her division, department, or institution.

There are, of course, constraints on the power of this position. The Director's role should be to help the various unrelated medical users in getting their diverse jobs done. Clearly, funding for medical research is granted on the merits of individual studies: The Director has no control over setting the budget for various projects and should have no power to usurp funds that were allocated for some other purpose. The Director of Clinical Computing may be responsible for several physical installations, ranging from simple computer-based instruments to large time-sharing systems. While encouraging users with similar interests to band together in shared facilities when it is in their best interest to do so, the Clinical Computing Director must recognize that primary responsibility will be to individual users or to *voluntary* associations of users. One approved and funded application cannot be held back because another unrelated project has failed to obtain adequate support.

The Director's responsibility for budget is to try to arrive at realistic estimates of cost, and to assist in efforts to persuade those who control the purse strings that these costs are necessary.

The Computer Advisory Committee

Pure research applications have no requirement for hospital service funding to achieve their primary project goals. Whether or not these projects succeed or fail is strictly a matter between the researcher and the funding agency.

However, when medical-computing applications are designed for rendering some service to patients, there is an overlap of interest between a clinical computing group and hospital administration. This overlap is best dealt with through a body that might be called the "Computer Advisory Committee," made up of representatives from both clinical and administrative computing departments, and of members of the various clinical departments and of the administration of the hospital. Examples of applications subject to such mixed management include admitting/discharge/transfer systems, patient registration schemes, radiology reporting systems, laboratory reporting systems, and so on. The committee setup involves the physicians and medical-computing experts who are responsible for the selection and/or development, implementation, and daily operation of computer services for patient care; and the hospital administrators who have responsibility for the efficient running of the service departments and who will have to find the means of paying for the development of the systems.

When a medical-computing project combines research and service goals, the Computer Advisory Committee should review the project to clarify the implied partnership of the hospital with the research funding agency. The project should be considered service-related to the extent that the hospital is required to finance it. The research-related aspects of the project should be clearly delineated, and it should be made clear that the institution will assume no financial liability for them. On the other hand, the service-related aspects should be considered in the same light as the pure service applications we have just considered.

The User's Role

If the Computer Advisory Committee is somewhat like the "Board of Directors" in a medical-computing application that directly concerns the institution, the Users' Committee might be analogous to the "stockholders." Users have an important role to play as a pressure group that lobbies to make sure that its own legitimate interests are met.

In hospital business computing, input from the comptroller, accountants, and administrative and junior management personnel will be important in identifying areas in which automation ought to be considered. Often, financial reasons are the primary motivating influence for undertaking a data processing application in business. However, nonmanagement personnel such as the clerical staff should not be forgotten, since they are often the people who will have to use a computer system with their own hands. Their perception of existing problems in the current method of performing any administrative function and their desire for improvement are very important. It is interesting to consider how often it happens that only the clerks truly understand the detailed mechanics of any business procedure, be it issuing checks or taking care of personnel records. Managers often do not know exactly how the processes work, even though they may have a global idea of what is going on.

In clinical computing applications concerned entirely with medical research, a somewhat different situation exists. Here it is the individual who is the motivating influence. The computing goals of medical research often require less of a cooperative effort than the kinds of business data processing seen in hospital administration. After all, it is the individual researcher who obtains funding for individual projects. If a project has been reviewed and approved through the proper channels of peer review, the researcher should be able to request and to obtain those computer services for which money has been approved. Therefore, the role of the Director of the clinical computer group is to assist the researcher in achieving project goals — not to direct the research or to hinder it in any way.

One of the best ways in which the medical-computing expert can assist researchers is by helping them to make the most of their rather limited financial resources. Computers are expensive, and usually any one researcher cannot obtain enough money for adequate hardware acquisition and software development. Hence the motivation for shared computer facilities and development. When possible, the person in charge of the facility should limit reinvention and thus enable the researcher with a new project to make use of hardware and software that is already developed or possibly underutilized. Equipment, development effort, and cost can thereby be contained at the relatively low level with which most research projects can cope. When new kinds of hardware must be acquired or new software developed, the director of the clinical computing group in question will be able to set realistic budgetary goals and to direct these new developments in such a way that they will benefit future users as well as current ones. This kind of cooperation under one unified management is essential if many little research projects requiring medical-computing services are to succeed at all.

The voluntarily cooperating association of users who agree to pool their resources must have a means of expressing collective priorities and desires. They do this through the Users' Committee, which should meet regularly.

THE FACTS OF LIFE

Today it is a fact of life that computing in the medical environment must to some extent be decentralized. The needs of medical research computing are so radically different from ordinary business data processing functions seen in the administrative sphere that these two kinds of computing cannot be combined. Their managerial philosophies, objectives, and fundamental hardware and software requirements are often mutually incompatible.

Within the clinical computing sphere it is a further fact of life that multiple physical installations are going to proliferate. Increasingly, computer-based medical instruments are appearing on the market that are totally self-contained. When development of a totally new system is undertaken, it is utter folly to attempt to combine some kinds of disparate applications such as signal processing and database management. Different kinds of systems are required to support these completely unrelated areas; programmers with different sets of skills are required for each. When requirements cannot be comfortably integrated, nothing but trouble will ensue if one tries to force them into a shotgun marriage. (See Chapter 2.)

At the same time, the average medical research application has such a small budget that separate acquisition of facilities is impossible in many circumstances. The economic necessity of pooling resources and avoiding duplication whenever possible makes it incumbent upon users with *compatible* requirements to band together in Users' Groups.

When medical computing is to be invoked as a means of delivering health care to patients, some method of effective management must be worked out so that all of the parties with a legitimate interest in the project can be represented.

Establishing effective management is the key to success. A successful implementation does not occur haphazardly. Its course is charted, and it is skillfully piloted under the command of one director through the shoals of budget, schedule, varying levels of user enthusiasm, and ever-changing requirements to its completion.

Organizing for automation is just as important as finding the right hardware and obtaining the proper software. Only when responsibility is unambiguously assigned and only when managerial authority is clearly delegated can one hope to avoid wasting valuable energy in internal political squabbles.

In this section we have seen that good management is as much a part of medical computing as computer hardware or software. It seems unfortunate, therefore, that many of the people who must fill the vacuum of managerial authority in medical computing have not had any specific training to prepare them for their jobs. Recent innovations at some universities would appear to support the belief that medical computing is a distinct profession with discernible demands and challenges, for which an appropriate academic curriculum should and can be devised.

Therefore, in the following chapter we will look more closely at the kind of training that could best prepare someone for a career as a medical-computing specialist.

NOTES

1. F. P. Brooks, *The Mythical Man-Month: Essays on Software Engineering.* Reading, Mass.: Addison-Wesley, 1975.

2. S. A. Glantz, Computers in clinical medicine: a critique. *Computer* 11:5:68, 1978.

EDUCATIONAL ISSUES

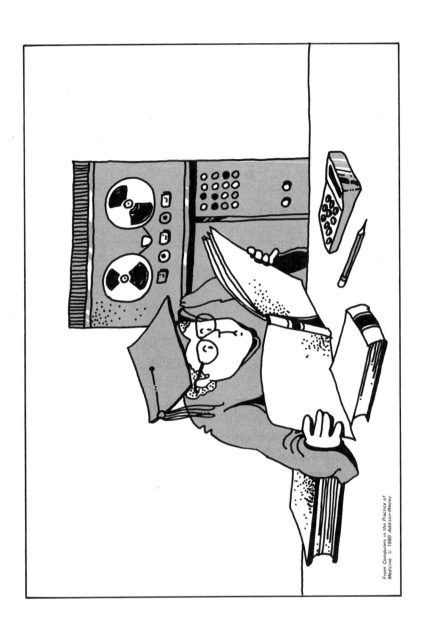

10

Training Medical-Computing Specialists

It may sound like a truism to say that the expertise of a graduate in computer science is in computer science, but the point is worth emphasizing. Business has long appreciated the fact that a computer science graduate seldom knows enough about the business environment to be useful without additional business-oriented academic and on-the-job training, because substantial differences exist between what is taught in a computer science department and what business data processing requires. For example, although COBOL is eschewed as a rather dull and cumbersome programming language in the academic environment, it still remains *the* principal programming language in the business community.

However, it is not only the computing details that differ between academic computer science and the computer science of the business world. Naturally, businesses are especially interested in accounting — a fact reflected in their data processing needs. Accountancy is not normally studied by computer scientists. Indeed, the entire framework of modern business, from its organizational methodologies to its basis in economics and the profit motive, has very little in common with the academic scene. Computer science is not likely to teach its students about the *kind* of information that will be required from a management information system or, for that matter, about how to apply such a system effectively — even if it does teach them about information systems!

Business, then, needs data processing services that are directed to its particular needs. As such, a commercial enterprise would probably hire a person holding a Bachelor's degree in computer science and a Master's degree in business administration (if they could find such a person) in preference to a Ph.D. in academic computer science. Innovation in computer science is usually not what interests business.

The academic community has responded to the needs of business by instituting in some business schools a strong computer science curriculum that is specifically directed to business applications.

Compared to business, the health-care system is a Johnny-come-lately to data processing, and the successful use of computers in medicine has not generally been perceived as being dependent on people who are knowledgeable in both computer science and medicine. The medical environment presents computer professionals with unique problems that their training usually does not anticipate. Previous experience with the business community will not greatly help these professionals either. Hospitals are like businesses in the sense that they are big institutions composed of many different departments. But they are unlike businesses in several important respects.

For one thing, the degree of autonomy exercised by each department within a hospital is generally greater than one might expect to find in a business enterprise of similar size. Whereas in businesses the profit motive is the overriding consideration that all departments must respect, in hospitals (especially in a socialized economy) there may be no such motivation. Different hospital departments frequently come into direct conflict with each other as they compete for the same dwindling supply of dollars. Their conflicts will often be resolved on other than a profit-related basis. The high degree of departmental independence is not confined to interdepartmental rivalry: It is fair to say that there is not even a true employer-employee relationship between most medical institutions and the physicians who work in them. Frequently the physician in a hospital works under a complex financial agreement in which fee-for-service plays a part. Each doctor is therefore his or her own boss to some extent — an observation underlined by the difficulty that our health-care institutions have in merely enforcing the completeness of their medical records! Establishing any kind of cooperative medical-computing venture in such an environment challenges diplomatic and administrative skills.

On the assumption that it is possible to get agreement in principle for a medical-computing venture, financing such a venture is uniquely frustrating in the health-care environment. A business need only satisfy itself that a piece of equipment or a procedure will save money or increase revenues in order to justify its use. In medicine, however, only some hospitals share such motivation. In Canada, for instance, the socialized form of medicine places hospitals under tight financial constraints, often precluding the expenditure of large amounts of money now in order to save more later. Even increased efficiency in dealing with a particular kind of medical problem can be interpreted negatively, since this simply means that more of such cases would be treated, with *increased* overall costs to the government!

Even when money can be found for medical computing, the computer scientist's frustrations are far from over. The very structure (when there is a structure) of medical decision making is inscrutable. The computer scientist called upon to implement useful computer-based systems in support of medical objectives is often required to invent the models on which to base programming. If physicians have not been able to elucidate a general approach for the evaluation and treatment of broad classes of patients, the computer scientist will obviously have trouble in doing so. At the very least, the computer scientist soon discovers that many problems are not computer-related, but rather that they involve the clarification, explication, and formalization of medical processes themselves.

THE SKILLS OF THE MEDICAL-COMPUTING SPECIALIST

In order to meet the unique challenges of applying data processing techniques to the medical environment, a person will require a combination of computer science training and some background in medicine. Such an individual will also need an understanding of areas that fall somewhere between the two disciplines but that are generally not dealt with in either one of them.

Computer Science Background

The medical-computing specialist will have a sound background in computer science. This person must have theoretical and practical knowledge of hardware and software, a good grasp of operating systems and compilers, and an understanding of modern database management systems (an area that is becoming more and more important in medical applications). Excellent knowledge of computer graphics and a minimum of one course in artificial intelligence are also important. At the applications programming level, the medical-computing specialist should have experience in a variety of programming languages and techniques, and at least one course in software engineering. This person's knowledge would not be complete without training in the economics of computing; a course or experience in the management of software development would also be preferred. In short, this person is expected to be a better-than-average computer scientist, *not* merely a "programmer." His or her salary will reflect this fact.

Medical Background

Those who will direct the development or the application of computers in medicine must have knowledge of the specific problem areas in which their computer system will be used. For example, a basic understanding of hospital administration is essential in the development of an admission/discharge/transfer system. Those who work on automated radiology reporting systems have to know about the problems that radiologists encounter and that automation might reasonably be expected to solve. The same analogy holds for every other application area in health care. Most of the time physicians will be quite unable to think about problems specific to their specialties in an organized, analytical way, nor will they be able to state these problems clearly enough to permit automation to proceed on either a rational or a practical basis. It will be the responsibility of the medical-computing expert to uncover and clarify these problems and to evaluate the potential role of computers in solving them. To do this, the computer scientist must be thoroughly integrated into the medical environment and must be completely at home with health-care personnel. When doctors use the medical jargon of their respective specialties, the medical-computing specialist must know what they are talking about.

There are a number of ways in which a non-health-care professional can obtain some familiarity with the medical environment. Perhaps one of the best ways is for such a person to undertake an apprenticeship under the tutelage of someone who is already expert in a particular medical-computing area, and who has already become very familiar with the particular medical problems under consideration. An additional useful approach to the medical education of a computer scientist would be the reading of appropriate books about clinical decision making, physiology, and the like. Those who need more in-depth knowledge in a particular area might be able to arrange to study or audit specific basic science courses in a medical school.

Those working in teaching hospitals will have access to a wealth of rounds and formal lectures in specific subject areas (such as cardiology, for example), some of which may be very useful.

Non-health-care professionals should not underestimate their own abilities to master selected areas of basic science that pertain to specific special-interest areas in medical computing. For instance, the physiology programs that are taught in the early years of most undergraduate medical programs can be profitably attended by anyone who has ever been exposed to university biology.

In addition to an overview of the medical environment at the departmental or specialist level, medical-computing people must acquire some understanding of the economics of health-care systems. A global view of the health-care system will assist the computing expert when he or she is called on for an opinion regarding the difficulty, expense, and priority of various possible medical-computing applications.

Special Training

Some of the background of the ideal medical-computing specialist cannot be obtained from a university computer science course, medical training, or immersion in a medical milieu.

Generally speaking, managerial skills make or break a computing venture. In business, data processing managers are trained on the job as they rise through a business hierarchy. In medicine, however, data processing is generally "small potatoes": Installations are small, and computer-knowledgeable staff are correspondingly few. Salaries are generally not competitive with buisness, so the turnover of computing staff in medical institutions tends to be high. It is therefore difficult for medicine either to attract high-level data processing managers as replacements or to retain the services of those who have received on-the-job training. This situation is unfortunate (and we hope temporary), because the degree to which a medical-computing project meets its goals on time and within budgetary constraints is determined to a huge extent by the management skills (or lack of them) of the medical-computing specialist.

Most computer science curricula teach virtually nothing about the nuts and bolts of acquiring computer equipment and services in the real world. However, a data processing manager obviously has to know about the selection of systems in the marketplace. He or she must be familiar with existing products and their comparative strengths, weaknesses, and prices. Similarly, an appreciation of the reputations, past records, and relative competence of various companies providing hardware and software services should be an integral part of a data processing manager's knowledge base.

A grasp of the economic issues of data processing in the real world includes familiarity with contracts, leases, rental agreements, and software maintenance and hardware maintenance agreements. The manager will require familiarity with all the arcane terminology of these contracts, so common to business.

The medical data processing manager needs to cultivate associations with the sales representatives of various companies. Most of these men and women are honest, decent people, whose principal objective is to serve their customers with the most appropriate products that their respective companies have to offer. However, some people are inherently more knowledgeable, or more hard working, or simply easier to get along with than others. A good working relationship with the local sales "reps" can be a decided asset to any data processing manager.

An additional and vital aspect of the training of a medical-computing specialist should be the review of previous medical-computing applications and the analysis of why they have either succeeded or failed. Some good general lessons can be learned from critical evaluation, and such an education may save a future practitioner of medical computing from wasting time on an insoluble problem or from trying to "invent" what could be bought over the counter. Often a course or two providing an introduction to medical computing are available at larger universities, and even more in-depth courses (on the application of database systems to medicine, for instance) are sometimes available. Taking such courses periodically as "refreshers" is a good idea in order to become familiar with what is going on in the outside world of medical computing.

Once equipment has been obtained and software has been acquired or developed, the medical-computing specialist must then *manage* a data processing application. Setting a budget (and sticking to it), establishing a schedule (and meeting it), guiding implementation, and supervising staff are no mean tasks. They require technical know-how, incessant vigilance, meticulous organization, and even diplomatic finesse.

Finally, good public relations between computer personnel and the medical community can be realized only by genuine understanding and goodwill on the part of both computer science types and health-care personnel. The medical-computing specialist as a person should exemplify this cooperative spirit, since he or she will be the most visible proponent of computer services in medical applications.

UNIVERSITIES MEET THE CHALLENGE

Institutions of higher learning are becoming aware of the unique skills required by the medical-computing expert. An increasing number of them are responding to this need by establishing courses or even whole curricula specifically directed towards educating people to fill this role. In general, two approaches have been taken: degree programs in medical informatics, and supplementary education in medical computing for graduates of other programs.

Degree Programs

Some universities have chosen to establish separate institutes granting degrees in medical informatics or medical information processing. These academic institutes are often hybrid organizations combining a variety of personnel from other academic areas such as computer science, medicine, biomedical engineering, and industrial engineering. The precise composition of such interdisciplinary institutes varies from place to place. The purpose of such institutes is, in general, two-fold. First, students in the institute receive specific training in medical information processing. Often only graduate students are accepted. Admission requirements may include degrees in either computer science or in medicine. Second, the institute serves as a liaison between the medical community and computer scientists. Ideally, it would be a resource for advice on the development of everything from a simple data entry form to an entire project. Advice

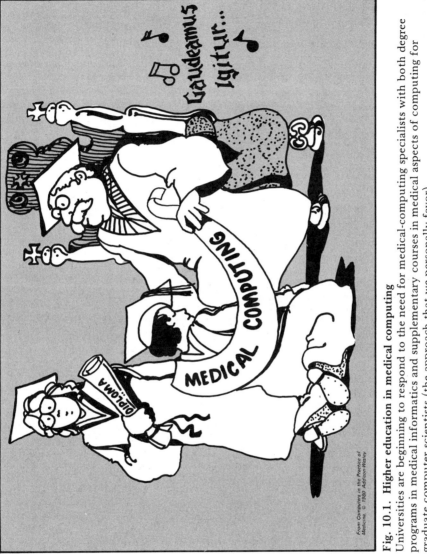

From Computers in the Practice of
Medicine. © 1980 Addison-Wesley

Fig. 10.1. Higher education in medical computing
Universities are beginning to respond to the need for medical-computing specialists with both degree
programs in medical informatics and supplementary courses in medical aspects of computing for
graduate computer scientists (the approach that we personally favor).

Table 10.1. Universities with Degree Programs in Medical Informatics

Duke University
Georgia Institute of Technology
Hunter College (New York)
Stanford University
University of California — San Francisco

regarding the selection or development of hardware and software might also be available from such an institute.

Table 10.1 lists those universities offering such an approach to medical information processing that replied to our inquiries by January 1979.

Supplementary Courses

A second kind of response by the academic world to the challenges of medical computing is in the approach that we personally favor: supplementing existing curricula in computer science with additional courses provided by other departments to qualify a computer science graduate as a specialist in medical computing. This approach seems less redundant than establishing a separate institute of medical informatics with a wide variety of courses that partially overlap those already being offered by the computer science department. Indeed, medical-computing experts ought to have the benefit of the best possible training in computer science, and it must be conceded that the most qualified teachers of computer science are to be found in that department. Introductory courses in "medical computing" are necessary, *but by no means sufficient,* to train a medical-computing expert. In-depth knowledge of computer science is mandatory. There is nothing to be gained and much to be lost by usurping the educational role of computer science departments that already handle this aspect of education very well.

The supplementary courses should concentrate on the knowledge that will transform a computer scientist into a *medical* computing expert. Biomedical engineering, medicine, industrial engineering, business administration, and computer science itself are departments that could individually or collectively offer some of these courses.

Table 10.2 Universities with Some Courses in Medical Computing

Baylor University
Bowling Green State University
Case Western Reserve University
Duke University
Georgia Institute of Technology
Johns Hopkins University
St. Louis University
Texas Tech University
University of Chicago
University of Florida — Gainesville
University of Southern California
University of Toronto

Table 10.2 lists those universities in North America that offer such supplementary courses in one or more departments. (These are the institutions that replied to our inquiries by January 1979.)

Examples of such courses are: the economics of medical computing, medical decision making, database systems in medicine, medical image processing, organization and management in health-care systems, product evaluation and selection, and many specialist-oriented courses (computers in cardiology, radiology, laboratories, administration, etc.).

Regardless of which approach a university may take to the training of medical-computing experts, an essential part of this training should take place in the medical environment. The "ivory tower" is not the place to learn about the practical needs and frustrations of computing in health care. Students must get out into the medical community to conduct their term projects, systems analysis assignments, and theses on a practical level. Encouraging such participation can only be to the advantage of the medical personnel with whom such projects will be carried out.

CONTINUING EDUCATION: KEEPING UP

A sound academic background is a firm foundation on which to build a career in medical computing. In order to maintain knowledgeability in the field, a medical-computing expert will need to keep abreast of ongoing developments.

Specialist Journals

A number of scholarly journals are devoted entirely to medical computing. These journals, a partial list of which is shown in Table 10.3, offer editorials, review articles, and individual project reports.

Books

The books written about certain aspects of medical computing are slowly increasing in number. We conducted a survey of numerous publishers in North America and Europe in 1978 (although our survey was not exhaustive). A list of the books we found was included as an appendix to *Computers in the Practice of Medicine: Introduction to Computing Concepts, Vol. I,* in this Addison-Wesley series on medical computing.

Medical Journals

Other publications in the medical literature (not specifically devoted to medical data processing) occasionally offer review articles or articles concerning specific applications in the medical-computing area. A MEDLINE search of the *Cumulated Index Medicus* shows that in 1976 and 1977, over 2500 articles concerned with some aspect of computers or automation appeared in the medical literature alone.

Other Technical Journals

Nonmedical technical literature such as the publications of the Association for Computing Machinery (ACM), or the Institute of

Table 10.3. Journals Devoted to Medical Computing

Computers and Biomedical Research
Computers and Medicine (AMA)
Computers in Medicine and Biology
Computer Programs in Biomedicine
Engineering in Medicine and Biology Society Newsletter (IEEE)
Health Communications and Informatics
International Journal of Biomedical Computing
Journal of Clinical Computing
Medical Informatics
SIGBIO Newsletter (ACM)

Electrical and Electronics Engineers (IEEE), occasionally publish interesting review papers about some aspect of computers in medicine. These publications are also very useful for maintaining an up-to-date knowledge about computer science in general.

"Trade" journals in data processing frequently provide excellent review articles about computing machinery and software practices, written by acknowledged experts in their fields. *Datamation* and *Mini-Micro Systems* are two such journals.

Symposia and Conferences

Several important meetings about medical computing take place regularly, and the proceedings of these conferences are required reading for anyone who wishes to know about the state of the art. The Medinfo International Conference occurs every three years. Annual conferences include Computer Applications in Medical Care, which covers a wide range of medical-computing interests; the Canadian Organization for the Advancement of Computers in Health; and Computers in Cardiology, which focuses on that specialty area. A partial list of other symposia and conferences is shown in Table 10.4.

Medical conferences are increasingly providing a platform for scientists who are using computers in an innovative way to advance medical knowledge. In addition, some of them have sponsored tutorial sessions about the use of computers in relevant specialty

Table 10.4 Symposia and Conferences

Artificial Intelligence in Medicine
Canadian Organization for the Advancement of Computers in Health
Computer Applications in Medical Care
Computers in Cardiology
Computers in Ophthalmology
Health Care Management and Informatics
Medcomp (International Conference on Computing in Medicine)
Medical Informatics in Ambulatory Care (International Conference on Medical
  Informatics)
Medinfo
Society for Computer Medicine
World Association for Medical Informatics

---

areas. The annual meetings of the American Heart Association, the Radiologic Society of North America, the Canadian Cardiovascular Society, and others have provided tutorials in computing. Similarly, other medical specialties have their own annual meetings, the proceedings of which may from time to time contain some important papers on the use of automated techniques.

Most of this reading material is available in libraries of computer science or medicine. Almost all of it is available by private subscription, although prices are usually high. However, some excellent trade journals such as *Datamation* are circulated without charge to a restricted list of qualified applicants: Fill out an application and see if you qualify.

Human Interaction

Reading alone is not likely to provide the intellectual stimulus to keep up with medical computing. It is just as important to remain involved in a project or with an institution where things are going on. By continuing interaction with others, one acquires new ideas, new viewpoints, and new techniques.

Attendance at one or two conferences per year is an excellent and enjoyable way to meet new friends and associates and to learn from them.

In addition, membership in societies and special interest groups is strongly recommended. Organizations such as the ACM and the IEEE have special interest groups with their own newsletters, meetings, and workshops.

GETTING STARTED

Students increasingly have the opportunity to obtain specialized training in medical computing. However, such opportunities did not exist even a few years ago, and they are still available only at a small number of universities. Therefore, many of the people who are now working as medical-computing specialists or who will be thrust into such a role in the near future will have to possess the initiative to obtain basic and/or continuing training for themselves.

The doctor, computer scientist, or hospital administrator who is becoming involved in medical computing is probably best advised to start gradually, with appreciation of the fact that he or she will have to spend *some* money on self-education.

It would perhaps be wise to form an informal liaison with a local university's computer science department. Get to meet one or two of the professors and discuss the plan you have in mind in a "brainstorming" session. It may be that the project that you propose is exciting enough to be the basis for a project for one or more computer science graduates or undergraduates. (Professors are always looking for practical projects for their students; the students, in turn, are gratified when their work is useful to somebody besides themselves.)

Would-be medical-computing experts can improve their knowledge about computer science by reading journals, symposia, books, and specialized publications. Even those physicians or hospital administrators who may have studied some computer science as undergraduates may be shocked at the progress that has taken place within the past decade, if they have not kept up with modern developments.

It would be worthwhile for those health professionals interested in medical computing to attend specialty conferences in their own field at which tutorial sessions on data processing are offered.

At a deeper level of commitment, a physician, hospital administrator, laboratory technologist, medical records librarian, head nurse, or other health-care worker with an interest in some aspect of medical computing could audit a course or two on the subject at a nearby university. Finally, those who wish to gain a working knowledge of medical data processing may be able to arrange a sabbatical in the laboratory of some specialist in this field. Six months or a year will not transform a health professional with inadequate computer science training into a medical-computing consultant, but it will at least enable such an individual to approach medical-computing applications with some confidence and basic knowledge of the many factors involved in securing their success.

Lastly, everything that we have said about continuing education for medical-computing specialists would apply to those who must teach themselves something of this discipline.

THE MEDICAL-COMPUTING SPECIALIST

Increasingly, we may see physicians, degree nurses, and hospital administrators taking postgraduate university work in medical informatics, as they recognize the finite commitment necessary to obtain a useful background in this subject.

However, the average health-care worker has such limited experience in computer science that he or she will seldom make good the deficiency. It is our belief that in the future, medical-computing specialists will hold a Bachelor's degree in computer science and probably a postgraduate degree of some kind, reflecting additional training in the medical aspects of computing. The growing number of universities responding to the challenge of medical computing with formal courses and curricula points the way to the future.

Although few of the health-care workers who will become end-users of medical-computing systems will ever become real medical-computing specialists, all will benefit from increased knowledge. Appreciation of the issues involved in medical computing, an understanding of the problems facing medical-computing specialists, and knowledge of the ways in which they should deal with these problems will greatly enhance users' chances of obtaining the computer services that they really require.

Therefore, in preceding chapters we have looked at the technical issues facing medical-computing projects. In this chapter, we have considered the kind of background and training that a medical-computing specialist ought to have — as much for the enlightenment of the health-care workers who rely on their services as for the education of those who wish to become expert in this field.

However, there is one further aspect of user training that should be considered: how to recognize, face, and conquer The Big Sell. The user's education as a *consumer* of medical-computing goods and services cannot be neglected. This is the subject to which we now turn our attention in Chapter 11.

BIBLIOGRAPHY

Canadian Organization for the Advancement of Computers in Health, Graduate education in computer systems in medicine. *Medical Informatics* 3:3, 1978.

11

Conspicuous Computing

Consumer Education

Even if only few of us are intimately familiar with the many remarkable things that computers have made possible, others are at least aware that computers have made possible many remarkable things. We are not saying these things are necessarily good: Those of us who have ever tried to explain to a creditor's computer that it has made a mistake know differently. Nevertheless, a suitably tamed computer is generally acknowledged (however reluctantly) to be a tangible manifestation of the progress and the ingenuity of humankind.

Computers are making inroads into health care, and their technical applications are abundantly discussed in a variety of publications. But the sociology of computing in the medical environment is seldom considered. We believe that, quite apart from any scientific or economic consideration, not the least of the factors responsible for the increasing use of computers in medicine is the same kind of motivation that makes people buy cars — not for transportation but for self-aggrandizement.

In recent years, consumer education has done much to draw the buyer's attention away from promotional gimmickry in the auto industry and toward practical considerations such as fuel economy and safety features. Similarly, the would-be consumer of medical-computing products and services would be well advised to seek education about the traps that are set for potential buyers in today's marketplace. Let us therefore look more closely at some of the pitfalls.

THE BAIT

Our society believes religiously in science as a source of knowledge and truth. Apart from a few heretics who are suspicious of anything scientific, most people — especially those who fancy themselves to be scientists — believe that science is a good thing and that just about everything associated with it represents progress and improvement. The revered offspring of science is technology, which we can loosely define as the implementation of the lessons of science.

The technological imperative — the compulsion to do things simply because they can be done — seems to be a motivation acquired during absorption in the beatific goodness of technology.

The computer is one of the most awesome incarnations of technology. It is incredibly complicated. It is fast beyond imagination. It is powerful and mysterious. It is even difficult to conceptualize, because it is a tool and yet not one that we can physically wield. Computers are remote and cannot be approached except by priestly technicians who speak their strange languages. Many computers are housed in inviolable temples called "Computer Centers," where none but the elect may enter.

A mystique therefore surrounds the computer and everything that it touches. In a society that adores technology it is perhaps inevitable that a great need to use computers whenever possible is felt — most notably in scientific professions such as medicine.

If you feel the call, then you're ripe for conversion. If you don't feel it, do not doubt that there are "missionaries" to entice and exploit you if you are a potential computer user. The techniques that they use are sales gimmicks that we all disdain, but to which we all seem to be susceptible in spite of ourselves. [1] Glossy three-color brochures featuring sexist pictures of shapely women flood the mailbox of the most casual inquirer. (See Figs. 11.1a and 11.1b.) Salespersons will flock to your door at the drop of a business reply card. Computers are styled with the precision of Detroit's latest chariot to turn your head and rivet your attention. (See Fig. 11.2.) Colors are picked with care. Dozens of idiot lights of no use to anyone but a repair person are prominently displayed because they look so nifty. Boxes housing microchips are larger than necessary because big is impressive. The price, economy, and real necessity of a computer system seldom figure in the sell. There is subtle emphasis not on what the computer can do for you, the user, but on what it can do for your image. You will be enticed to identify self-betterment with the product. The product will be presented as something by which you may acquire characteristics that you could not otherwise possess. The pitch to your ego can be irresistible, as common experience proves. People who once sold us big fancy cars convinced us that by buying them we could show the world how successful we

See what you're missing... it's time to ask for a sample of "Vision One" quality image processing: the first choice of specialists.

By definition, an *image* is the digitally stored representation of the shape and shadings of objects, people or scenes. And, *processing* is the enhancement of brightness, color and definition of the image.

Printed reproductions cannot do justice to the quality of Vision One Image Processing Systems. To see what you're missing, send to Comtal for samples of Vision One image quality and standard interactive processing features.

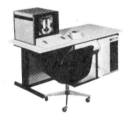

Vision One is delivered ready to operate on digitized imagery without a host system/software development or time-consuming software installation or integration.

Vision One is an intelligent image processing system featuring real-time, completely operator interactive image processing for black and white or full 24-bit color (8 bits each of red, green and blue). Image resolution is 256x256, 512x512, or 1024x1024 pixels with internal solid state memory for up to fifteen 512x512 images (8-bit) and sixteen 512x512 graphic (1-bit) overlays.

Comtal is the acknowledged leader in digital image processing and offers the first commercial system with these features:

Real-time roam of multiple displays in very large data base memories (1977), stand-alone image processing systems, real-time small area independent color correction, and real-time convolution processing (1975). Also, 1024x1024, 256 shade soft-copy display image processing system (1974), full 24-bit color and digital image function and pseudo-color image processing (1973), with single standard digital interface for all features and options (1972).

Comtal has the only commercial systems with real-time operator interactive image processing and hardware generated display of image processing test patterns.

Fig. 11.1a. A woman's place?
What the male chauvinist readers see is supposed to persuade them to like what they can't see. There may be many good reasons for selecting this product — but the pretty model is not among them. (The authors wish to acknowledge the permission given by the COMTAL Corporation for use of their advertising material in this book.)

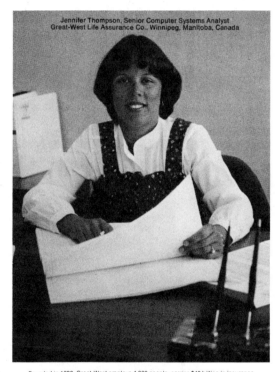
Fig. 11.1b.
Fortunately, times are changing. Although some technical details about this product may have changed since this ad appeared in December 1978, the attitude toward women expressed here is progressive, modern, and entirely nonsexist. (Reprinted by permission of Informatics Inc.)

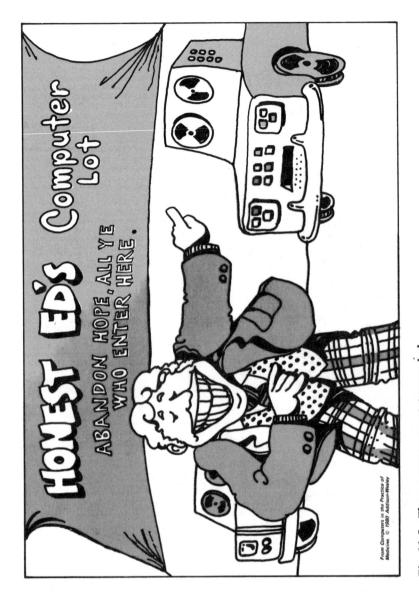

From Computers in the Practice of Medicine. © 1980 Addison-Wesley

Fig. 11.2. The computer as a status symbol
Computers are styled with the precision of Detroit's latest chariot to turn your head and rivet your attention!

were. Now, responding to consumer pressure, they have cleverly learned to sell us half the car (for the same money) so that we can flaunt self-images of common sense, "thrift," and conservation-mindedness. Diabolical! The truth is unimportant when you, the customer, can be taught to *believe* in the transforming power of a product: You are not drinking soda pop — you are partaking of the Fountain of Youth!

THE HOOK

So with computers. Our health facilities are filled with the same gullible consumers that our homes are. Physicians and administrators are right now being wooed by clever advertising designed to create needs not previously felt. They are told to believe that computers can do great things for them and their images — even by their own professional associations.

Conspicuous computing! The computer is that vital element separating plain arithmetic from higher mathematics. It transforms a common laboratory into a hotbed of innovation, dignifies ordinary record keeping with the mantle of "database management," and changes mere dabbling into a research project. Above all, computing elevates you above your colleagues. Your aura of power at scientific gatherings waxes fat. The very presence of such expensive equipment in your department is irrefutable evidence of your authority and influence. Yes, the person who has a computer is a person to be reckoned with.

So speak those who push computers on potential medical users. They actively foster the "mark's" fond conceit that computerization will herald a new era — a veritable "quantum leap" for the organization or department.

THE STING

Too often it is a leap into space. Without knowing precisely why he or she wants a computer, driven by a desire to be better and by an enthusiastic belief in technology, the prospect becomes a customer. We say "belief" because, under existing conditions, acquiring a computer is often an act of faith. A small computer can cost as much as several cars, and most computer systems are more expensive than a house. However, there are no Ralph Naders, no Better Computing Bureaus, and often not even a lawyer automatically hired to uphold your end of a deal in a contract — if there ever is a contract. *Caveat emptor* never applied more strongly than to the buyer of a computer. Yet the same consumers who would demand guarantees for the functioning of a $50 coffeemaker are remarkably trusting when spending huge amounts of other people's money on a medical-computing system!

Computer advertising promises products that work. It assures the consumer that a particular system will solve specific problems. Sometimes a buyer gets such a product — for example, in an instrument such as a CT scanner in which the built-in computer functions as part of a larger machine. The built-in computer's purpose is well defined and its functional performance is guaranteed so that buying this product is like buying a car. Generally, though not always (with apologies to Flip Wilson), "what you see is what you get."

The same *can* be true of a prefabricated "turnkey" computer system that is supposed to do your work as soon as you plug it in and turn it on. Some examples are radiology reporting systems, monitoring systems, admitting/discharge/transfer systems, cath lab data acquisition systems, and the like. The computer system here is intended to *be* the instrument — not just to be a controller *in* the instrument, as in the CT scanner.

But a computer system is truly an instrument only to the extent that it is a useful, consumable product. The danger here is two-fold. First, the "general" system, designed as a solution-to-everyone's-problem, may not fit *your* specific needs, and getting the company that supplies it to do the modifications may be difficult. Second, some systems are put together almost in a way analogous to assembling the parts of a kit: computer from here, software from there. To continue the automobile analogy, this approch is like buying a crate full of parts in order to convert your Volkswagen into a dune buggy. The advertising shows a picture of the finished product, but if you assemble the vehicle and it doesn't run — tough bananas! You took the responsibility. You get the headaches.

If you purchase the wrong kind of computer instrument, or if you inadvertently assemble a computer monster, there are only two options open: You can either get rid of the computer or you can change your entire department to fit the system such as it is. The latter approach at least spreads the suffering around. There are many places you can visit to see how this is done, but self-preservation keeps us from being specific.

At a stratum of complexity above turnkey systems are computer systems that do not even pretend to be finished products. Let's call them general purpose systems. For one example, a system for hospital database management is a highly complex and hard-to-pin-down entity. To use the automobile analogy again, what you acquire is the whole assembly line. You will need analysts, programmers, and keypunchers to design, tool-up for, assemble, and test whatever the final product may be. Here you must be extremely careful and you must get professional help.

The ultimate danger is not merely failure: The financial stakes can be high. The remains of once grandiose medical-computer schemes lie de-energized in the back rooms of our institutions, attesting to the significant mortality rate of medical-computing projects.

DON'T BE A MARK

Disaster can occur if one proceeds solely on the pitches of people intent on providing bits of computer tinsel to grant-fattened crows. So avoid being motivated by the little blinking lights and the sexist ads. Don't swoon at the thought that "computerization" will metamorphose you into the Bionic Health-Care Worker. Remember that you may be the victim of seduction!

Educated consumers of computing products and services aimed at the health-care market will know what they want and what they are getting into. Their knowledge can save them from being gullible "marks" for sharp salespersons and can help them to get the kinds of systems that they really need.

In the long run, knowledgeable consumers will be a boon not only to themselves and to the agencies that ultimately bear the cost of medical computing, but to the data processing industry also. No businessperson wants to fight with dissatisfied clients — it is simply bad business. From all points of view, then, the best customer is an educated consumer!

NOTE

1. P. Crabtree, and R. Kling, Data processing sales ploys and counterploys. *Datamation* 25:5:194 (May) 1978.

SUMMING UP

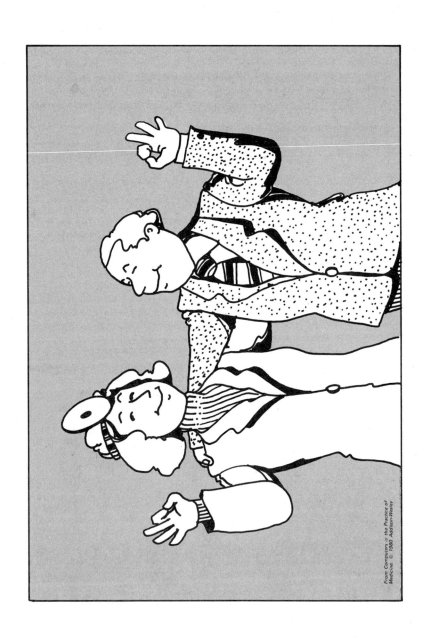

12
Funding Medical Computing

Applying For Money

Medical research projects and "pilot projects" testing innovative methods of health-care delivery cost money. When computers play a part in such projects, they are often a significant cost component. Health-care workers who want to undertake expensive work of this sort can obtain funding from a variety of sources. A rich person or one who needs only minimal computer services may be personally able to foot the bill for something like an office computer. However, in most cases it will be necessary to find external revenues.

Whether approaching his or her own department or an agency for money, the health-care worker will have to convince peers that the proposal is sound. (See Fig. 12.1.) A written document is normally the vehicle in which an applicant delivers arguments to those who will decide the fundability and therefore the life or stillbirth of the project. A proposal for a computer system to be used in a medical environment can be constructed in such a way that it anticipates and answers convincingly most of the pointed questions that a referee might have. The model proposal will demonstrate that the applicant has considered every one of the critical issues in medical computing and is thus no optimistic amateur. It will further illustrate that the advocate of the proposal has realistically anticipated potential problems and therefore has a good chance of surmounting them.

A PLAN FOR A FORMAL PROPOSAL

A general plan for the presentation of a formal proposal for a medical-computing system is shown in Table 12.1. A document approximately corresponding to such a plan would be quite suitable for application for funding from most agencies. Naturally, the precise form will have to be modified somewhat in accordance with the requirements of the various agencies that are approached, but we can examine generally most of the parts that such a document should contain.

I. Summary

The first part of the document might be considered an "abstract" of the rest. In technical proposals, this section is often called

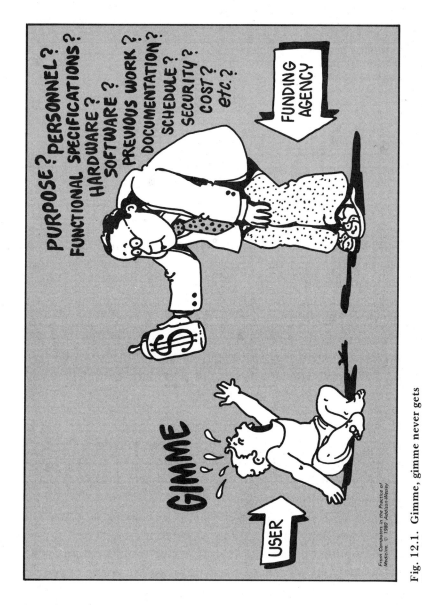

Fig. 12.1. Gimme, gimme never gets
You seldom encounter a sucker in a funding agency these days. When you're in competition with other scientists, you've got to convince the people who control the purse strings!

Table 12.1. Parts of a Model Grant Application

     I. Summary
    II. Introduction to the problem
   III. Functional specification (précis)
    IV. Previous work
     V. Critical analysis/comparison
    VI. Selection or plan
   VII. Economic analysis
  VIII. Schedule
    IX. Operational detail
     X. Appraisal of system
    XI. Appendices
        A. Relevant publications
        B. Existing systems to choose from
        C. Functional specification (details)

the "Executive summary." In not more than five pages devoid of technical jargon, the salient facts of the proposed project should be stated in such a way that those unfamiliar with the field of medical computing can understand the essence of what is being proposed and its total cost.

It sometimes happens that a referee is so busy that there will only be time to read this summary: Therefore, this section must be concise, clear, and informative. *It may be the most important section of the entire proposal.*

II. Introduction to the Problem

In this section, the problem for which automation is proposed as a solution should be stated and then detailed. Dissect the problem area into component parts and make considered judgments about what parts of the problem will be easy or difficult to solve.

This section would be a good place to demonstrate that you have considered alternative solutions to your problem that do not call for a computer. The reasons why each alternative will not work should be stated. (If you cannot state such reasons, why are you talking about an expensive computer system?)

For research projects, experimental method and justification for the anticipated outcome are obviously fundamental components of any application for funding. It is the responsibility of the applicant to provide this information in the context of his or her field of research.

When a computer system is proposed as a tool for carrying out a scientific research project, the use of this (probably expensive) instrument will have to be justified. If a small fee for performing a few statistical calculations on a computer system is proposed, there should be no problem. However, at the other extreme, when the computer system itself is the subject of the research — for instance, when an automated information management system is proposed as part of a novel method of health-care delivery — adequate information must be included in the proposal to demonstrate to reviewers that the approach is sensible and potentially successful.

III. Functional Specification

Functional specifications have already been explained extensively in Chaper 6. At some point in the formal proposal, you should state the kind of automated solution that is required to deal adequately with the problem(s) outlined in the previous section. If it is decided to concentrate only on some big, fairly straightforward problem areas and to deliberately avoid small but knotty problems, the functional specification should reflect this choice. This section states *what* you want the proposed system to do when it is installed and working.

The functional specification is a complex statement reflecting broad understanding of many of the issues that have been discussed. In addition to the ultimate expected performance of the computer system, other related issues such as security (which will also be part of your solution, whatever you decide) must be addressed. It is quite possible to relegate the details of the functional specification to an appendix in order to make the overall document more readable.

If your proposal is approved, then this section — the functional specification — will serve as a guideline for suppliers when you request quotations from then. Finally, it will be incorporated with modifications into a contract.

IV. Previous Work

This section demonstrates that the person making the proposal has done the necessary homework and is intent on avoiding reinvention in cases in which development is proposed. First, there must be a review of the literature about previous similar work (if any). Include a list of specific references. If there are few or even no such references, document the fact and state how this conclusion was reached. If there are one or two particularly relevant review articles, it is often wise to include reprints of them as appendices to this document.

If there are acknowledged experts in the field under consideration or people who have successfully completed somewhat similar work, include their names, addresses, and telephone numbers if you can. This attention to detail will make the referees' work easier for them.

There may be computer products available commercially to perform the kind of work that you are contemplating. For example, if you were proposing the acquisition of an automated coronary care unit monitoring system, you should indicate in your proposal that you are aware of the numerous commercial systems available for the purpose and that you have evaluated each one of them carefully. It will suffice to identify these commercial products in this section and to list the companies that supply them, together with the names, addresses, and telephone numbers of local representatives of those companies. The salient features and quoted prices for all of the commercial systems mentioned in this section should be included as another appendix to the entire document. It would not be reasonable to include in the body of the document a detailed analysis of many possible systems, only one (if any) of which will ultimately be proposed.

V. Critical Analysis/Comparison

In this section, you should compare the functional specifications to the work that has previously been done at other centers or to the presently available commercial products (turnkey systems).

The purpose of this section is to whittle down the field to a list that includes only those products or previous projects that are capable of meeting the functional specifications you have stipulated. If there is no existing work that would suit your purposes, state that fact here and indicate that you intend to develop a new system or tailor one to your needs.

VI. Selection or Plan

If you can use a commercially available computer system or a system that you can buy or copy from some other center, specify your choice in this section.

It may be necessary to modify an existing product so that it matches the functional specification. If you take this approach, assess the feasibility and cost of such changes.

On the other hand, you may get to this stage and find that for the sake of simplicity or for economic reasons, you should modify your functional specification to match one of the available products! If this is your honest conclusion, it may be better to go back and change your original functional specification accordingly. If you get this far before deciding that your original goals were impractical, you should rethink the entire project before submitting your proposal for peer review.

If there is no existing system capable of meeting your functional specification, then substitute for this section your plan for developing your own unique system. State whether you will be establishing your own in-house data processing team or whether you intend to hire outside developers. Give an accurate impression of the size of the proposed operation and the general length of time that you expect development to take. (Note section IX below.)

VII. Economic Analysis

We have already dealt with the problems of an economic analysis in fair detail. At this point in your proposal, you should enumerate the current and projected costs of implementing the automated solution that you selected in the previous section. The issue of cost-benefit should be formally defined in your document for the sake of readers who are not familiar with this term, and you should then break down your analysis in detail. Similarly, you would probably be well-advised to define cost-effectiveness before attempting to make some kind of analysis of this rather fuzzy issue. Remember that very few people have *ever* demonstrated a computer system to be clinically effective at anything by any quantitative criterion. Referees are not likely to be impressed by pious claims of "improved quality of medical care" in the absence of compelling arguments or evidence to this effect.

VIII. Schedule

State the schedule for the development, testing, and implementation of the proposed system.

Indicate how you intend to monitor the performance of the development team. What landmarks are to be used? What is the schedule for achieving these landmarks? The schedule for testing and debugging the system, for installing it on your premises, and for running it in parallel with manual procedures, together with the date on which you plan to commit exclusively to automated methods, should be listed.

IX. Operational Detail

This section of the proposal should discuss how the computer system will be managed on a day-to-day basis, once it is operational. The overall process in which the computer may be only one cog should be outlined, and the computer's role in this process should be detailed. How will the computer impact on the people using it and on the way they do business?

Equally important is consideration of how quality control of the automated system would be ensured. For example, it is relatively easy to define a data collection system in support of clinical trials: It is difficult, on the other hand, to guarantee that data essential to the success of the research will be collected and input to the computer system correctly. [1]

X. Appraisal of System

How will you know whether or not your computer system has achieved the goals you set out for it? What are the acceptance tests that must run correctly before you will accept the system from a developer? How will you recognize failure if it occurs, and what will you do to cut your losses if necessary? It has often happened that a computer system directed to a specific purpose has seemed like a good idea in the proposal, but has been unworkable in the implementation. Given such experience, it only makes sense for the applicant to leave open reasonable escape routes. There is nothing shameful about an honest experiment that ends in honest failure. Indeed, this kind of experience may serve as a valuable lesson to future workers in the area. On the one hand, it is reprehensible to close one's eyes to the possibility of failure or to refuse to acknowledge it when it occurs, since this will waste everyone's money, time, and effort.

XI. Appendices

The three appendices already mentioned (relevant survey articles, analysis of available systems from which to choose, and the details of the functional specification) will be included at the end of the application for funding. In addition, any other relevant appendices that do not logically belong in the body of the text can be included here.

Generally speaking, one is well advised to keep the body of any document as thin and to-the-point as possible. Referees do not have much time to wade through an inch-thick stack of paper. They want to get at the bare facts of the proposal and to be secure in the knowledge that further details, documentary evidence, and the like are available in appendices if required.

CONCLUSIONS

It is desirable to structure an application for funding in the previously outlined way for two reasons. First, a well-planned and persuasively stated proposal is much more likely to evoke a favorable response than a vague request for lots of money and the trust of the granting agency. Enlightened self-interest should be motivation enough for the would-be user of medical-computing systems to accept this somewhat compulsive format.

But the second reason for making an organized, thoughtful proposal goes far beyond personal interest. Society can no longer sanction the wanton expenditure of large sums of money on questionable medical "research" or flashy medical gadgetry. The mere perception that computers are supposed to be modern and progressive does not qualify them for use in the medical environment. They are costly and difficult to employ intelligently, and when misused, they can have a deleterious influence on health care. Those who would embark on a course that involves automation therefore have a responsibility to consider all the issues implicit in a move toward medical computing, and a proposal such as the one outlined here helps the person originating a computer project to remember all the issues.

The effort required to produce such a document is considerable, but it is worthwhile. Those who make the effort and who know enough about medical computing to perform the task adequately may be satisfied that they are proceeding in an informed, reasonable, ethical manner. Their goals, their reasons for using computers, their logic in making their selection, and the financial implications of their proposals will all be laid out plainly, so that their peers can also make a reasonable, informed decision.

It is impossible to know with certainty where automation will lead the healing arts. The benefits that medicine may reap from computers may be limited only by our imagination. But the potential dangers — financial and ethical — are sufficiently plain that everyone who works in this expanding field has a personal obligation to keep both eyes open. No good and much harm may derive from the blind pursuit of "progress" through technology. Everyone who proposes, designs, or uses computer systems in the health-care environment must understand the issues underlying medical automation.

Only through our continuing efforts to cope with all the implications of the grand new technology at our disposal can we determine whether computers will be abused as agents of dehumanization in the most human of our arts, or whether computers will be incorporated as our faithful servants.

NOTE

1. I. K. Crain, Entry and validation of scientific data: how to prevent "garbage in." *INFOR* 15:160, 1977.

13
Quo Vadis?

The Future of Medical Computing

Since the days of the Delphic Oracle (who was at least smart enough to couch her predictions in ambiguous terms so that she would be right whatever happened), soothsayers seem to have lost their classical touch. Some modern swamis, economists, and government representatives are dismally inaccurate in their rosy predictions about the future.

However, in regard to computers, the pundits may actually have been too cautious in their visions of a glorious future.

Twenty years ago, ambitious engineering students and faculty sometimes built their own computers at great expense and with hundreds of hours of effort. The home-brew computers that these pioneers developed were just novelties. They could not be programmed easily, and once programmed, they often could not save the program for later retrieval on a mass storage device. The output of these machines was usually restricted to binary displays of lights. These interesting projects in electrical engineering were done to try new ideas and to gain experience — not usually to support an application as mundane as business or medicine.

However, today the situation has changed beyond the wildest dreams of even the visionaries of the last decade. For less than a hundred dollars, one can purchase a basic, programmable calculator that performs arithmetic, trigonometric, some algebraic, and even statistical functions. The low price includes a rechargeable battery, a charger, and a carrying case. For less than $400, one can purchase a programmable calculator similar in physical size, but with the ability to store many hundreds of programming steps and with a mechanism to save programs on magnetic strip cards for later use. Firmware read-only memory modules, providing preprogrammed packages for applications such as statistics or accounting, can be purchased separately and are plugged into the back of the calculator as required.

Today we are even able to obtain complete microprocessor-based systems (with disks, tape, and terminals) that are far more powerful than the computers of yesteryear, but whose price is less than a single terminal was in those days.

Twenty years ago, these commonplace realities would have seemed like fantasies. Since the modern computer reality has so richly outdone the most optimistic predictions of its advocates, it would not be entirely unreasonable for us to imagine that the future impact of computers on medicine may be bound only by man's imagination and not by technical limitations. Based on that admittedly speculative hypothesis, what might one be able to predict about the future of automation in medicine?

WHY TO USE A COMPUTER SYSTEM IN MEDICINE

How computers serve medicine will always depend on our insights into their relevance and on how we choose to use them. We can now already distinguish several important roles for computers.

Personnel Augmentation

Computer systems can be used to augment human resources wherever there exists a tested, working, and proved manual process whose capacity it is necessary to expand, whose speed it is necessary to increase, or whose repetitive parts it is desirable to unload from people. A computer properly integrated into such a situation can enhance the efficiency of existing personnel so that they can handle an increased workload more easily or an existing workload more quickly or less expensively. Computer systems used in such situations would have to be less expensive than hiring additional people to cope with the increased workload, and they should not decrease the overall "effectiveness" or usefulness of the procedure. Preferably, the computer should enhance the environment it becomes a part of and not dehumanize it.

To illustrate how computers can enhance the roles of humans within an organization, let us consider how a fully automated cardiac pacemaker registration system could operate in a "typical" big hospital.

With labor costs such as they are, it had been found costly to maintain active, long-term followup on every patient who had ever received a cardiac pacemaker in our hypothetical large hospital. Frequent followup of cohorts of patients with similar types of pacemakers was out of the question. Consequently, the standard procedure for replacement of a pacemaker was either to wait until it started to malfunction and the patient got into trouble, or to replace an implant long before it was expected to wear out. Either way, the situation was undesirable. However, today all recipients of cardiac pacemakers have been registered on a computer-based system for several years. Patients who have had pacemakers can telephone at regular intervals, and by placing simple-to-use electrodes under their arms, they can transmit a rhythm strip to the computer over the telephone. The computer notes if there is any impending malfunction in the pacemaker and issues warning letters to the patient and the physician as required. It has thus been possible to prolong the useful life of a pacemaker implant, thereby saving not only money but a good deal of inconvenience and surgical morbidity for the patients. Moreover, when it is discovered that a particular kind of pacemaker is failing prematurely, it is a simple matter to locate and recall all patients with similar equipment for prophylactic replacement. This feat would have been impossible without some kind of up-to-date centralized registry. Thus, computers can be used in the Pacemaker Clinic to tangibly enhance the clinical effectiveness of the existing clinic staff: They can now anticipate and prevent emergencies, rather than merely respond to them. Patient care has been improved.

A completely automated system such as the one described here could be implemented by simply combining features of partially automated pacemaker followup systems already in existence throughout the world.

Management Augmentation

When an existing process is soundly conceived, useful, efficient, but very tedious or complex, maintaining and managing that process may be difficult. The amount of paperwork involved in documenting and ensuring that all steps in a complicated procedure are carried out may be burdensome. In such cases, computers can serve a "policing" or disciplinarian role, because these machines are capable of mindless perseveration on even the most tedious and boring details of a management process. Dull and repetitive aspects of management can be handled by the computer. Moreover, the system can measure parameters of performance and provide such information to management, so that various aspects of a complex process can be quality-controlled or modified as required for increased efficiency.

As an extension of management augmentation, a computer can be used to initiate a very complicated process that because of its intricate and consequently expensive management requirements could not be implemented in any other way. In such cases the computer is used as the framework on which a new process is built.

One good example in medical research is using a computer to manage clinical trials. Accurate and complete patient identification and documentation, as well as continuous monitoring of the data collection process, can reduce the cost of carrying out trials with a significant decrease in the effort necessary for quality control.

Brain Augmentation

An ideal use of computers is to augment the human's ability to handle information and to make decisions. Computers can perform feats of calculation, information storage and retrieval, and data manipulation that would be out of the question to accomplish manually.

An extension of this capability is the use of computers to simulate processes in order to refine our understanding of a phenomenon. Physiological and biochemical models are two examples relevant to medicine. Similarly, a computer can be used to model a complex procedure, in order that we may study the inherent time delays, costs, and bottlenecks.

In the near future, we might expect significant advances in computer-aided diagnosis and decision making. These are essentially modeling problems, and as we gain more insight into the ways in which physicians approach clinical management, it will become increasingly more possible to assist them in this process by using computer-based models.

WHY NOT TO USE A COMPUTER SYSTEM IN MEDICINE

We have examined general roles for computers in medicine both now and in the future. However, computers are sometimes proposed or actually used for reasons whose justification defies discernment. One would hope that in the future we would be able to avoid what we might call "antiroles" of computers in medicine.

Robot "Physicians"

We believe that computers as we know them should not be used as a means of directly *treating* human patients without the supervision of human physicians — even if this remote possibility becomes technically feasible, as some people have predicted. [1] Computers must always be used to assist but never to replace the physician. Many of the decisions that a doctor must make have as much (or more) to do with the assessment of the emotional status of the patient and the perception of the patient's willingness to endure treatment as they do with purely technical matters. The warmth, concern, perception, sensitivity, and compassion that are integral to the healing arts may never be replaced by technology, and those who attempt to do so are ignorant of the capabilities of our systems and of our inherent lack of understanding of human processes.

Self-Aggrandizement

Because computers are expensive, and because their implementation has a drastic impact on all users, these machines are potentially disruptive tools, subject to abuses of local political power. Disaster is the result when hospital administration, one medical department, a clique, or an individual has a stranglehold on data processing within an institution through the control of a centralized computer facility and/or its development staff. However, this admonition is not made to advocate a completely *laissez-faire* attitude. Those who crave technology as a means of demonstrating scientific "leadership" or of otherwise impressing their colleagues can waste a great deal of other people's time, effort, and money, once they perceive the computer to be the most prestigious vehicle for an ego trip. As automation makes ever greater inroads into the medical scene, all concerned parties must beware of people who want computers for various kinds of self-aggrandizement. (See Fig. 13.1.)

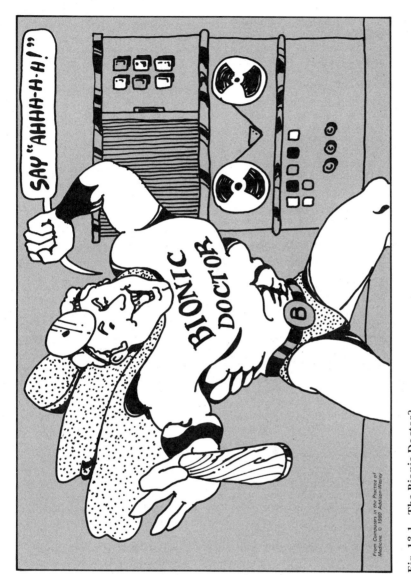

Fig. 13.1. The Bionic Doctor?
Hardly! Automation will play a beneficial role in the future of medicine — but only if we use it wisely. Those who seek computers for self-aggrandizement should find other toys. (Drawing adapted [with apologies!] from M. Harrison, L. McCartney, and R. McLaughlin. Captain COBOL. *Datamation* 24:4:148 (April) 1978.)

Supporting Obsolete Methods

A common abuse of computers is to use them to prolong the life of dying lines of evolution in management practice. State-operated health insurance may be a case in point. Some existing centralized systems are too large to adequately serve the people who depend on them. In one Canadian province, for instance, it is estimated that there are more employees working for the provincial health insurance plan than there are physicians in the whole province. The fact that the government is unwilling to release precise figures on this matter tends to confirm the suspicion. The system is characterized by enormous operating expenses, [2] frequent delay of payments for 60 days or more, and even occasional mysterious payments to physicians for services they have neither rendered nor claimed! The system is inefficient and technically obsolete. It could not long continue without computer support.

If there were no computers, such unmanageable centralized schemes would be replaced by a network of much smaller local offices that would be able to process their business in a more timely and efficient manner, probably with less danger of making mistakes and with more potential for assisting in the correction of errors.

Although health care is no longer the "growth industry" that it once was, it will continue to grow in the future. We should beware, lest computers be used to prop up obsolete procedures in health-care administration when decentralization or innovation is really indicated.

Robbing People of Work

There is a risk, not only in medicine but in all types of business, that in the future, computers will take over more and more of the interesting and challenging aspects of work, leaving only boring "watching the gauges" functions to people. We would hope that in the future, medicine will avoid using computers merely to replace human beings unless significant cost savings and/or *measurable* improvements in health-care delivery can be effected by so doing. In other words, automation should proceed not by blind compulsion, but only through necessity.

Enshrining the Theoretical

Whenever a computer system is used in the medical environment in the future, let us hope that it is used in accordance with proved, well-thought-out principles.

Because computers require the quantizing and simplification of reality into discrete parameters that can be measured, stored, retrieved, and processed, there will always be a danger that they will be used to oversimplify reality, especially when the original conception of reality is faulty. Computers do just what we tell them — the ultimate embodiment of the "we only followed orders" personality. All the thinking had better be done by people *before* they bring a computer into the picture.

A PROMISING FUTURE

If computers were to be applied in health care to exploit their positive aspects, and if medicine could avoid their potentially bad features, then the future of medical computing might be rosy indeed. Let us try to imagine where computers in medicine are going.

Hardware Advances

First of all, they are going out of sight — and ultimately, out of mind. The trend in computer hardware is toward miniaturization. This trend will probably continue. At present, computers or their peripheral devices are still far too large to be truly convenient. To succeed as commonplace, everyday instruments, they will have to become less obtrusive and more portable. We can expect that the current generation of rather clumsy computer teminals will be refined immeasurably, so that they can become as easy to use as pocket dictaphones, for instance. This development would do much toward making the computer input device at least as usable as a pencil, because it would improve the accessibility and abundance of computer terminals.

Computer systems in medicine will become more justifiable on purely economic grounds because they will become cheaper, and therefore they will become more common in everyday medicine. Microprocessor technology has already drastically influenced the design and the cost of computer hardware, but this effect may yet be only the tip of the iceberg.

The coming years should see the success of computer-controlled devices that can be implanted in the human body. As the machinery of computers becomes smaller and smaller, computers will be able to become parts in more elaborate instruments such as "intelligent" pacemakers, artificial limbs, and perhaps someday, even artificial organs — except, perhaps, the brain. It is not at all difficult to imagine that miniaturization of computer hardware and the development of new power sources and transducers will soon make the Bionic Man a matter of commonplace experience, not of science fiction.

Leaping to the furthest bounds of imagination, one can imagine that a means will be found to interface computers with the human nervous system. Such an advance would make possible the creation of artificial eyes, ears, and voice generation.

Intelligent, implantable devices that are capable of measuring such variables as heart rate, rhythm, and blood pressure could automatically infuse antiarrhythmic drugs to control arrhythmias, for instance.

Implantable devices containing a computer could also be used beneficially in high-risk patients. For instance, an implantable device might be designed for patients with a history of severe heart disease. When the computer detected a dangerous arrhythmia, it could automatically "dial" an ambulance to take the patient to a hospital. This kind of device is almost realizable today: The communications technology and the computer itself already exist. Here, the big limit is in understanding arrhythmias: When they have been understood, the develoment of appropriate control software will be possible. This area will undoubtedly be the subject of intensive research in the near future.

Advances in digital communications and storage devices will also have a profound influence on the use of computers in medicine. The ideal of a "cradle-to-grave" medical record is presently impossible, given the mobility of our population and the relative expense and awkwardness of communications facilities. However, as it becomes cheaper and easier to transmit volumes of data over wide distances, the distributed database in medical records could become a reality.

Another approach to the lifelong personal medical record may be a record that patients carry with them wherever they go. It is not difficult to conceptualize a tiny storage device that could be implanted in a patient's body (subject, of course, to the patient's approval!) with no side effects whatever. At a hospital there would be a device for reading this history and for updating it as required.

Software Advances

Software development will keep pace with advancing hardware technology. Perhaps at some time in the future we may actually look forward to computer systems that can respond to "natural language" in the form of typed input or even in the form of speech. Similarly, computers themselves may learn to speak to us in our own language, to "speak" as we do, [3] and to interpret drawings and pictures as easily as we can. The overall trend in the future should be toward less arcane computer systems that ordinary people can use effectively with little prior training. Although far more pervading, computers will become infinitely less conspicuous.

In graphics, computers as parts of computed tomography instruments have already been used to show physicians what their own eyes cannot see. We will soon have graphical computer output in three or more dimensions. For example, one of these additional dimensions may be time. Computer-generated movies, though already impressive, are still in their infancy, and much more elaborate 3D (holographic) output is ultimately in the offing.

When hardware and software advance sufficiently, people will be able to interact with the computer more directly. Already patients can have their blood pressure checked by a machine in many supermarkets. Would it be unreasonable to predict that at some future date a patient may be able to undergo an automated routine checkup? The patient could converse with a computer that would ask relevant questions and listen to the spoken answers. Then the machine would make some biological measurements, using a few attached devices such as those to measure blood pressure, heart rate, ECG, and so on. These sorts of machines would be used principally for routine physical examinations. If anything significant were found, the patient would be instructed to see the human doctor. It has already been conceded that an annual routine physical examination for every citizen would be economically impossible. Computers might help make it possible — given the (admittedly questionable) assumption that there is a good reason for conducting such screening examinations of symptomless people.

In the immediate future, we would expect to see tremendous advances in the development of medical knowledge bases: systems to represent our understanding of pathologic processes and treatment strategies. By the use of sophisticated models, we will be able to test, check, and verify hypotheses with an ease not previously imagined.

Advances in Our Attitudes

As medicine learns to rely on the methods of systems analysis in order to employ computers most effectively where they are most needed, it may learn to use these and other analytical tools to study more objectively the things that are done in health care. Dogmas will be evaluated and empirical procedures will be increasingly questioned. The distressing tendency of the medical establishment to adopt as standard practice potentially hazardous investigations and treatments that have not passed any objective tests of efficacy or cost-justification may slowly come to an end as computers make large and complex evaluations of treatment and investigative procedures easier to carry out. Large cooperative studies have always been difficult to manage: Automation will undoubtedly simplify such studies and may thereby encourage them.

The computer has arrived on the medical scene at a time when physicians are becoming aware that clinical research ought to be a professional activity in its own right performed by medical scientists — not a mere sideline of medical practice. Computers may be one of the most powerful tools of future clinical researchers. Automation may thereby greatly reduce the reliance of medical science on the inconclusive case studies that have traditionally been conducted by part-time investigators. Computers may herald a new era in which demonstrable conclusions replace results that are merely sampling effects.

Automation may also help medicine to make a good adjust-ment to the problems induced via extreme specialization. The average patient is simply bewildered by the increasing compart-mentalization of medicine into specialties, subspecialties, and sub-subspecialties. [4] In fact, the average general practitioner is often no less confused. (Any specialist is well aware of the numerous inappropriate referrals he or she receives.) Any social worker is aware of the many patients whose welfare seems to fall between two or more stools, because each of several agencies assumes that somebody else is looking after the client. Every intern and resident knows that the more specialists involved in a case, the more likely something will go wrong. Automated systems may someday help general practition-ers and their patients to navigate through the increasingly complex maze of specialists, hospitals, and social services, making sure that the vital central factor — the patient — is not forgotten in the shuffle, that adequate records are kept, and that the quality of the overall process is maintained.

A POSITIVE INFLUENCE

Assuming that proper respect is paid to the practical issues in medical computing, there is every reason to suppose that automation will play a substantial and beneficial role in the future of medicine. If we use these machines to do the things that we cannot do without them, to help us do what we do not have time to do presently, and to encourage us to look at our medicine from a more scientific view-point, then we will be using computers appropriately, and we can expect maximum benefit from them.

It is how we choose to use automation that will determine its ultimate impact on the future of health care, for it seems probable that computer technology, like all the rest of technology, will ad-vance faster than we know how to use it in the service of humankind.

NOTES

1. J. S. Maxmen, *The Post-Physician Era: Medicine in the Twenty-First Century.* New York: Wiley, 1976.

2. E. L. Book, Problems of health insurance in Canada. *N. Engl. J. Med.* 298:1483, 1978.

3. J. L. Flanagan, Computers that talk and listen: man–machine communication by voice, *Proc. IEEE* 64:405, 1976.

4. L. D. Wilcox, *Where is My Doctor?* Toronto: Fitzhenry & Whiteside, 1977.

BIBLIOGRAPHY

Reiser, S. J., *Medicine and the Reign of Technology.* London: Cambridge University Press, 1978.

INDEX